Instructor's Manual

Dosage Calculations:
A Ratio-Proportion Approach

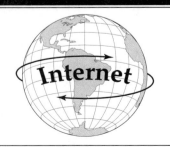

Instructor's Manual

Dosage Calculations: A Ratio-Proportion Approach

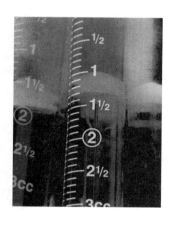

First Edition

Gloria D. Pickar, RN, EdD

Seminole Community College
Sanford, Florida

Prepared by

Beverly Meyers, BA, MEd

Jefferson College
Hillsboro, MO

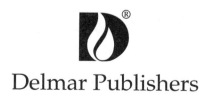

Delmar Publishers

an International Thomson Publishing company

Albany • Bonn • Boston • Cincinnati • Detroit • London • Madrid
Melbourne • Mexico City • New York • Pacific Grove • Paris • San Francisco
Singapore • Tokyo • Toronto • Washington

CONTENTS

Part 1   Answers/Solutions to Chapter Review Sets and Practice Problems

Mathematics Diagnostic Test (page 1)

1. 1517.00
    + 0.63
    ———
    1517.63

2. XIX + VIII = (19 + 8) = **27**

3. 9.50
    17.06
    32.00
    41.11
    + 0.99
    ———
    100.66

4. $19.69
    + $304.03
    ———
    $323.72

5. 93.20
    − 47.09
    ———
    46.11

6. 1005.0
    − 250.5
    ———
    754.5

7. 6003
    − 5995
    ———
    8 = **VIII**

8. 509
    × 38.3
    ———
    1527
    4072
    1527
    ———
    19,494.7

9. $4.12
    × 42
    ———
    824
    1648
    ———
    $173.04

10. 17.16
    × 23.5
    ———
    8580
    5148
    3432
    ———
    403.260 = **403.26**

11. $972 \div 27 =$ **36**

$$27\overline{)972}$$
$$\underline{-81}$$
$$162$$
$$\underline{-162}$$
$$0$$

12. $2.5 + 0.001 =$ **2500**

$$0.001\overline{)2.500.}$$
$$\underline{-2}$$
$$05$$
$$\underline{-5}$$
$$000$$

13. $176 + 16 = 11 =$ **XI**

$$16\overline{)176}$$
$$\underline{-16}$$
$$16$$
$$\underline{-16}$$
$$0$$

14. $1500 \div 240 =$ **6.25**

$$240\overline{)1500.00}$$
$$\underline{-1440}$$
$$600$$
$$\underline{-480}$$
$$1200$$
$$\underline{-1200}$$
$$0$$

15. $0.8 = \frac{8}{10} = \mathbf{\frac{4}{5}}$

16. $\frac{2}{5} = 0.4 \qquad 0.4 = \frac{4}{10} = \frac{40}{100} = \mathbf{40\%}$

$$5\overline{)2.0}^{\,0.4}$$

17. $0.004 = \frac{4}{1000} = \frac{0.4}{100} = \mathbf{0.4\%}$

18. $5\% = \frac{5}{100} = \mathbf{0.05}$

19. $33\frac{1}{3}\% = \frac{33\frac{1}{3}}{100} = \frac{\frac{100}{3}}{100} = \frac{100}{3} \div 100 = \frac{100}{3} \times \frac{1}{100} = \frac{1}{3} = \mathbf{1:3}$

20. $1:50 = \frac{1}{50} = \mathbf{0.02}$

$$50\overline{)1.00}^{\,0.02} \text{ or } \frac{1}{50} = \frac{2}{100} = \mathbf{0.02}$$
$$\underline{-100}$$
$$0$$

21. $\frac{1}{2} = \frac{2}{4}$
     $+ \frac{3}{4} = \frac{3}{4}$
     $\frac{5}{4} = \mathbf{1\frac{1}{4}}$

22. $1\frac{2}{3} = 1\frac{16}{24}$
     $+ 4\frac{7}{8} = 4\frac{21}{24}$
     $5\frac{37}{24} = \mathbf{6\frac{13}{24}}$

23. $1\frac{5}{6} = 1\frac{15}{18}$
     $- \frac{2}{9} = \frac{4}{18}$
     $\mathbf{1\frac{11}{18}}$

24. $\frac{1}{100} \times 60 = \frac{60}{100} = \frac{\cancel{6}^{3}}{\cancel{10}_{5}} = \mathbf{\frac{3}{5}}$

25. $4\frac{1}{4} \times 3\frac{1}{2} = \frac{17}{4} \times \frac{7}{2} = \frac{119}{8} = \mathbf{14\frac{7}{8}}$

$$\begin{array}{r} 14 \\ 8\overline{)119} \\ -\ 8 \\ \hline 39 \\ -32 \\ \hline 7 \end{array}$$

26. $\frac{1}{150} = 0.00666\ldots$

$$\begin{array}{r} 0.0066\ldots \\ 150\overline{)1.0000} \\ -\ 900 \\ \hline 1000 \\ -\ 900 \\ \hline 100 \end{array}$$

$\frac{1}{200} = 0.005$

$$\begin{array}{r} 0.005 \\ 200\overline{)1.000} \\ -1\ 000 \\ \hline 0 \end{array}$$

$\frac{1}{100} = 0.01$

$$\begin{array}{r} 0.01 \\ 100\overline{)1.00} \\ -1\ 00 \\ \hline 0 \end{array}$$

$\mathbf{\frac{1}{100}}$ is the fraction with greatest value, or, because numerators are the same, the fraction with the smallest denominator has the greatest value.

27. **0.009** has least value.

28. $\frac{6.4}{0.02} = \mathbf{320}$

$$\begin{array}{r} 320 \\ 0.02\overline{)6.40.} \\ -6 \\ \hline 0\ 4 \\ -\ 4 \\ \hline 00 \end{array}$$

29. $\frac{0.02 + 0.16}{0.4 - 0.34}$ $\dfrac{\begin{array}{r}0.02\\+0.16\end{array}}{0.18} \div \dfrac{\begin{array}{r}0.40\\-0.34\end{array}}{0.06}$ $0.06\overline{)0.18.} = \mathbf{3}$

30. $\frac{3}{12+3} \times 0.25 = \frac{3}{15} \times 0.25 = \frac{0.75}{15} = \mathbf{0.05}$

$$\begin{array}{r} 0.05 \\ 15\overline{)0.75} \\ -75 \\ \hline 0 \end{array}$$

31. 8% of 50 = $0.08 \times 50 = \mathbf{4}$

or 8% of 50 = $\frac{8}{\cancel{100}_{2}} \times \cancel{50}^{1} = \frac{8}{2} = \mathbf{4}$

$$\begin{array}{r} 0.08 \\ \times\ 50 \\ \hline 4.00 \end{array}$$

32. $\frac{1}{2}\% = 0.5\% = 0.005$

$$\begin{array}{r} 0.005 \\ \times\ \ 18 \\ \hline 040 \\ 005 \\ \hline 0.090 = \mathbf{0.09} \end{array}$$

33. 0.9% of 24 = $0.009 \times 24 = \mathbf{0.22}$

0.9% = $0.9 + 100 = 0.009$

$$\begin{array}{r} 0.009 \\ \times\ \ 24 \\ \hline 036 \\ 018 \\ \hline 0.216 \end{array}$$

34. $\frac{500}{125} = \frac{1.25}{X}$
     $500X = 156.25$
     $\frac{500X}{500} = \frac{156.25}{500}$
     $X = \mathbf{0.3125 \text{ or } 0.31}$

$$\begin{array}{r} 0.3125 \\ 500\overline{)156.2500} \\ -150\ 0 \\ \hline 6\ 25 \\ -\ 5\ 00 \\ \hline 1\ 250 \\ -1\ 000 \\ \hline 2500 \\ -2500 \\ \hline 0 \end{array}$$

35. $\frac{300}{150} \times 2 = \frac{600}{150} = 4$ or $\frac{\cancel{300}^{2}}{\cancel{150}_{1}} \times 2 = 2 \times 2 = 4$

$$\begin{array}{r} 4 \\ 150\overline{)600} \\ -600 \\ \hline 0 \end{array}$$

36. $\frac{5}{1.5} = \frac{2.5}{X}$
     $5X = 3.75$
     $\frac{5X}{5} = \frac{3.75}{5}$
     $X = \mathbf{0.75}$

$$\begin{array}{r} 0.75 \\ 5\overline{)3.75} \\ 3\ 5 \\ \hline 2\ 5 \end{array}$$

37. $\frac{\cancel{1,000,000}}{\cancel{250,000}} \times X = 12$
     $\frac{\cancel{100}^{4}}{\cancel{25}_{1}} \times X = 12$
     $4X = 12$
     $\frac{4X}{4} = \frac{12}{4}$
     $X = \mathbf{3}$

38. $\dfrac{1.7}{X} = \dfrac{0.51}{150}$

$0.51X = 255$

$\dfrac{0.51X}{0.51} = \dfrac{255}{0.51}$

$X = \mathbf{500}$

$$\begin{array}{r} 150 \\ \times\ 1.7 \\ \hline 105\ 0 \\ 150 \\ \hline 255.0 \end{array}$$

$$0.51\overline{)255.00}\quad \begin{array}{r} 500. \\ -255 \\ \hline 0\ 00 \end{array}$$

39. $X = (82.4 - 52)\dfrac{3}{5}$

$= (30.4)\dfrac{3}{5}$

$= \dfrac{91.2}{5}$

$X = \mathbf{18.24}$

$$\begin{array}{r} 30.4 \\ \times\ \ 3 \\ \hline 91.2 \end{array}$$

$$5\overline{)91.2}\quad \begin{array}{r} 18.24 \\ -5 \\ \hline 41 \\ -40 \\ \hline 1\ 2 \\ -1\ 0 \\ \hline 20 \\ -20 \\ \hline 0 \end{array}$$

40. $\dfrac{\frac{1}{150}}{\frac{1}{300}} \times 1.2 = X$

$\dfrac{1}{150} \times \dfrac{300}{1} = \dfrac{300}{150} = 2$

$2 \times 1.2 = X$

$2.4 = X$

$X = \mathbf{2.4}$

41. $2:10 =$

$\dfrac{\overset{1}{\cancel{2}}}{\underset{5}{\cancel{10}}} = \mathbf{\dfrac{1}{5}}$

42. $2\% =$

$\dfrac{2}{100} = \dfrac{1}{50} = \mathbf{1:50}$

43. 25 tabs : 5 containers = X tablets : 1 container

$\dfrac{25}{5} = \dfrac{X}{1}$

$5X = 25$

$\dfrac{5X}{5} = \dfrac{25}{5}$

$X = \mathbf{5\ tablets\ per\ container}$

44. 1 lb : 4 cups = X lb : 1 cup

$\dfrac{1}{4} = \dfrac{X}{1}$

$4X = 1$

$\dfrac{4X}{4} = \dfrac{1}{4}$

$X = \mathbf{\dfrac{1}{4}\ lb\ per\ cup}$

45. $\dfrac{66}{2.2} = 30$ or 1 kg : 2.2 lbs = X kg : 66 lbs

$\dfrac{1\ kg}{2.2\ lb} = \dfrac{X\ kg}{66\ lbs}$

$2.2X = 66$

$\dfrac{2.2X}{2.2} = \dfrac{66}{2.2}$

$X = \mathbf{30\ kg}$

$$2.2\overline{)66.0}\quad \begin{array}{r} 3\ 0 \\ -66 \\ \hline 0\ 0 \end{array}$$

46. 1 kg : 2.2 lb = 1.5 kg : X lb

$\dfrac{1\ kg}{2.2\ lb} = \dfrac{1.5\ kg}{X\ lb}$

$X = \mathbf{3.3\ lb}$

$$\begin{array}{r} 2.2 \\ \times 1.5 \\ \hline 110 \\ 22 \\ \hline 3.30 \end{array}$$

47. 1 cm : $\dfrac{3}{8}$ in = X cm : $2\dfrac{1}{2}$ in

$\dfrac{1\ cm}{\frac{3}{8}\ in} = \dfrac{X\ cm}{2\frac{1}{2}\ in}$

$\dfrac{3}{8}X = 2\dfrac{1}{2}$

$\dfrac{\frac{3}{8}X}{\frac{3}{8}} = \dfrac{2\frac{1}{2}}{\frac{3}{8}}$

$X = 6\dfrac{2}{3}$

$X = \mathbf{6.67\ cm}$

$2\dfrac{1}{2} \div \dfrac{3}{8} =$

$\dfrac{5}{\cancel{2}} \times \dfrac{\overset{4}{\cancel{8}}}{3} = \dfrac{20}{3} = 6\dfrac{2}{3}$

$$\dfrac{2}{3} = 3\overline{)2.00}\quad \begin{array}{r} .666\ldots \\ -1\ 8 \\ \hline 20 \\ -18 \\ \hline 20 \end{array}$$

48. $\dfrac{\$1.25}{\$0.25} = \mathbf{5\ quarters\ used}$

$$0.25\overline{)1.25.}\quad \begin{array}{r} 5 \\ -1\ 25 \\ \hline \end{array}$$

49. $\dfrac{5}{50}$ incorrect

$\dfrac{45}{50}$ correct

$$50\overline{)45.0}\quad \begin{array}{r} 0.90 \\ -45\ 0 \\ \hline 0 \end{array}$$

$0.90 = \dfrac{90}{100} = \mathbf{90\%\ answered\ correctly}$

50. **5:1**

Review Set 1 (page 5)

1. 28 = **XXVIII**

2. 13 = **XIII**

3. 17 = **XVII**

4. 15 = **XV**

5. $9 = \mathbf{IX}$

6. $VII + XXIII = 7 + 23 = \mathbf{30}$

7. $XXVII - IV = 27 - 4 = \mathbf{23}$

8. $XIX - XIV = 19 - 14 = \mathbf{5}$

9. $XII \times II = 12 \times 2 = \mathbf{24}$

10. $XXIV \div VI = 24 \div 6 = \mathbf{4}$

11. $5 \times 4 = 20 = \mathbf{XX}$

12. $18 + 12 = 30 = \mathbf{XXX}$

13. $16 \div 4 = 4 = \mathbf{IV}$

14. $625 \div 125 = 5 = \mathbf{V}$

$$125\overline{)625}$$
$$\underline{-625}$$
$$\;\;\;0$$

with quotient 5.

15. $17 + 14 - 11 + 4 = 24 = \mathbf{XXIV}$

$17 + 14 + 4 - 11 = 35 - 11 = 24$

Review Set 2 (page 8)

1. $\dfrac{6}{6}, \dfrac{7}{5}$

2. $\dfrac{\frac{1}{100}}{\frac{1}{150}}$

3. $\dfrac{1}{4}, \dfrac{1}{14}, \dfrac{1\frac{1}{4}}{14}$

Notice that the numerator of $\dfrac{1\frac{1}{4}}{14}$ is less than the denominator, so it is a proper fraction

4. $1\dfrac{2}{9}, 1\dfrac{1}{4}, 5\dfrac{7}{8}$

5. $\dfrac{3}{4} = \dfrac{6}{8}; \dfrac{1}{5} = \dfrac{2}{10}; \dfrac{3}{9} = \dfrac{1}{3}$

6. $6\dfrac{1}{2} = \dfrac{13}{2} \qquad \dfrac{(6 \times 2) + 1}{2} = \dfrac{13}{2}$

7. $1\dfrac{1}{5} = \dfrac{6}{5} \qquad \dfrac{(5 \times 1) + 1}{5} = \dfrac{6}{5}$

8. $10\dfrac{2}{3} = \dfrac{32}{3} \qquad \dfrac{(10 \times 3) + 2}{3} = \dfrac{32}{3}$

9. $7\dfrac{5}{6} = \dfrac{47}{6} \qquad \dfrac{(7 \times 6) + 5}{6} = \dfrac{47}{6}$

10. $102\dfrac{3}{4} = \dfrac{411}{4} \qquad \dfrac{(102 \times 4) + 3}{4} = \dfrac{411}{4}$

11. $\dfrac{\overset{2}{24}}{\underset{1}{12}} = \mathbf{2}$

12. $\dfrac{\overset{1}{8}}{\underset{1}{8}} = \mathbf{1}$

13. $\dfrac{30}{9} = 3\dfrac{3}{9} = \mathbf{3\dfrac{1}{3}}$

$$9\overline{)30}$$
$$\underline{-27}$$
$$\;\;\;3$$

with $3\dfrac{3}{9}$

14. $\dfrac{100}{75} = 1\dfrac{25}{75} = \mathbf{1\dfrac{1}{3}}$

$$75\overline{)100}$$
$$\underline{-75}$$
$$\;\;25$$

with $1\dfrac{25}{75}$

15. $\dfrac{44}{16} = 2\dfrac{12}{16} = \mathbf{2\dfrac{3}{4}}$

$$16\overline{)44}$$
$$\underline{-32}$$
$$\;\;12$$

with $2\dfrac{12}{16}$

16. $\dfrac{3}{4} \times \dfrac{2}{2} = \dfrac{\mathbf{6}}{\mathbf{8}}$

17. $\dfrac{1}{4} \times \dfrac{4}{4} = \dfrac{\mathbf{4}}{\mathbf{16}}$

18. $\dfrac{2}{3} \times \dfrac{4}{4} = \dfrac{\mathbf{8}}{\mathbf{12}}$

19. $\dfrac{2}{5} \times \dfrac{2}{2} = \dfrac{\mathbf{4}}{\mathbf{10}}$

20. $\dfrac{2}{3} \times \dfrac{3}{3} = \dfrac{\mathbf{6}}{\mathbf{9}}$

21. Because numerators are the same, the fraction with the smaller denominator has the greater value. So $\dfrac{1}{100}$ is larger, or,

$$150\overline{)1.000}\quad 0.0066\ldots$$
$$\underline{-900}$$
$$\;1000$$
$$\underline{-900}$$
$$\;1000$$

$\dfrac{1}{150} = 0.0066\ldots$

$\dfrac{1}{100} = 0.01$

$\dfrac{1}{100}$ **is larger.**

$$100\overline{)1.00}\quad 0.01$$
$$\underline{-1\,00}$$
$$\;\;\;\;0$$

22. Because the numerators are the same, the fraction with the larger denominator has the smaller value. So $\frac{1}{10,000}$ is smaller

$$1000\overline{)1.000}\quad\begin{array}{r}0.001\\-1\,000\\\hline 0\end{array}\qquad \frac{1}{1000}=0.001$$

$$\frac{1}{10,000}=0.0001$$

$$10,000\overline{)1.0000}\quad\begin{array}{r}0.0001\\-1\,0000\\\hline 0\end{array}\qquad \frac{1}{10,000}\textbf{ is smaller.}$$

23. $\frac{5}{9}$ **is larger.**

The denominators are the same. Fraction with larger numerator has larger value

24. $\frac{3}{10}$ **is smaller.**

The denominators are the same. Fraction with smaller numerator has smaller value.

25.

$\frac{1}{2}$ of $\frac{1}{4}=\frac{1}{2}\times\frac{1}{4}=\frac{1}{8}$

Each child's slice $=\frac{1}{8}$ of whole pizza.

26. $\frac{1\text{ bottle}}{12\text{ doses}}=\frac{X\text{ bottles}}{18\text{ doses}}$

$$12X=18$$

$$\frac{12X}{12}=\frac{18}{12}$$

$$X=\frac{18}{12}=\frac{3}{2}=1\frac{1}{2}\textbf{ bottles}$$

27. $\begin{array}{r}57\\+3\\\hline 60\end{array}$ people in class

The men represent $\frac{3}{60}$ or $\frac{1}{20}$ of the class.

28. $\frac{18}{20}=\frac{9}{10}$

29. $\frac{80}{160}=\frac{1}{2}$ **of a dose.**

30. $\frac{1}{2}$ of 1 teaspoon $=\frac{1}{2}$ **teaspoon.**

Review Set 3 (page 14)

1. $\frac{\overset{1}{\cancel{3}}}{10}\times\frac{1}{\underset{4}{\cancel{12}}}=\frac{1}{40}$

2. $\frac{12}{25}\times\frac{3}{5}=\frac{36}{125}$

3. $\frac{5}{8}\times 1\frac{1}{6}=\frac{5}{8}\times\frac{7}{6}=\frac{35}{48}$

4. $\frac{1}{100}\times 3=\frac{3}{100}$

5. $\frac{\frac{1}{6}}{\frac{1}{4}}\times\frac{\frac{2}{3}}{\frac{3}{2}}=\left(\frac{1}{\cancel{6}}\times\frac{\cancel{4}}{1}\right)\times\left(\frac{3}{1}\times\frac{3}{2}\right)=\frac{2}{3}\times\frac{9}{2}=\frac{\cancel{2}}{\cancel{3}}\times\frac{\cancel{9}}{\cancel{2}}=\mathbf{3}$

6. $\frac{\frac{1}{150}}{\frac{1}{100}}\times 2\frac{1}{2}=\frac{1}{\cancel{150}}\times\frac{\overset{2}{\cancel{100}}}{1}\times\frac{5}{\cancel{2}}=\frac{5}{3}=\mathbf{1\frac{2}{3}}$

7. $\frac{30}{75}\times 2=\frac{60}{75}=\mathbf{\frac{4}{5}}$

8. $\begin{array}{r}7\frac{4}{5}=7\frac{12}{15}\\+\frac{2}{3}+\frac{10}{15}\\\hline 7\frac{22}{15}\end{array}=\mathbf{8\frac{7}{15}}$ $7\frac{22}{15}=7+1\frac{7}{15}=8\frac{7}{15}$

9. $\frac{3}{4}+\frac{2}{3}=\frac{9}{12}+\frac{8}{12}=\frac{17}{12}=\mathbf{1\frac{5}{12}}$

$$12\overline{)17}\quad\begin{array}{r}1\frac{5}{12}\\12\\\hline 5\end{array}$$

10. $\begin{array}{r}4\frac{2}{3}+5\frac{1}{24}+7\frac{1}{2}=4\frac{16}{24}\\5\frac{1}{24}\\+7\frac{12}{24}\\\hline 16\frac{29}{24}\end{array}=\mathbf{17\frac{5}{24}}$ $16\frac{29}{24}=16+1\frac{5}{24}$ $=17\frac{5}{24}$

11. $\frac{3}{4}+\frac{1}{8}+\frac{1}{6}=\frac{18}{24}+\frac{3}{24}+\frac{4}{24}=\frac{25}{24}=\mathbf{1\frac{1}{24}}$

12. $\begin{array}{r}12\frac{1}{2}=12\frac{3}{6}\\+20\frac{1}{3}+20\frac{2}{6}\\\hline \mathbf{32\frac{5}{6}}\end{array}$

13. $\frac{3}{4}-\frac{1}{4}=\frac{2}{4}=\mathbf{\frac{1}{2}}$

14. $\begin{array}{r}8\frac{1}{12}=8\frac{1}{12}=7\frac{13}{12}\\-3\frac{1}{4}-3\frac{3}{12}-3\frac{3}{12}\\\hline 4\frac{10}{12}=\mathbf{4\frac{5}{6}}\end{array}$

15. $\frac{1}{8}-\frac{1}{12}=\frac{3}{24}-\frac{2}{24}=\mathbf{\frac{1}{24}}$

16. $\begin{array}{r}100\frac{1}{33}=100\frac{1}{33}=99\frac{34}{33}\\-33\frac{1}{3}-33\frac{11}{33}-33\frac{11}{33}\\\hline \mathbf{66\frac{23}{33}}\end{array}$

17. $355\frac{1}{5} = 354\frac{6}{5}$

    $\underline{-\ 55\frac{2}{5}\ -\ \ 55\frac{2}{5}}$

    $\quad\quad\quad\ \mathbf{299\frac{4}{5}}$

18. $\frac{1}{60} \div \frac{1}{2} = \frac{1}{\overset{}{\underset{30}{\cancel{60}}}} \times \frac{\overset{1}{\cancel{2}}}{1} = \mathbf{\frac{1}{30}}$

19. $2\frac{1}{2} \div \frac{3}{4} = \frac{5}{2} \div \frac{3}{4} = \frac{5}{\underset{1}{\cancel{2}}} \times \frac{\overset{2}{\cancel{4}}}{3} = \frac{10}{3} = \mathbf{3\frac{1}{3}}$

20. $\frac{\frac{1}{20}}{\frac{1}{3}} = \frac{1}{20} \times \frac{3}{1} = \mathbf{\frac{3}{20}}$

21. $\frac{1}{150} \div \frac{1}{50} = \frac{1}{\underset{3}{\cancel{150}}} \times \frac{\overset{1}{\cancel{50}}}{1} = \mathbf{\frac{1}{3}}$

22. $\frac{\frac{3}{4}}{\frac{7}{8}} \div \frac{1\frac{1}{2}}{2\frac{1}{3}} = \left(\frac{3}{\underset{1}{\cancel{4}}} \times \frac{\overset{2}{\cancel{8}}}{7}\right) \div \left(\frac{3}{2} \times \frac{3}{7}\right) = \frac{6}{7} \div \frac{9}{14} = \frac{\overset{2}{\cancel{6}}}{\underset{1}{\cancel{7}}} \times \frac{\overset{2}{\cancel{14}}}{\underset{3}{\cancel{9}}} = \frac{4}{3} = \mathbf{1\frac{1}{3}}$

23. $\frac{\frac{3}{5}}{\frac{3}{4}} \div \frac{\frac{4}{5}}{1\frac{1}{9}} = \left(\frac{\overset{1}{\cancel{3}}}{5} \times \frac{4}{\underset{1}{\cancel{3}}}\right) \div \left(\frac{\overset{2}{\cancel{4}}}{5} \times \frac{9}{\underset{5}{\cancel{10}}}\right) = \frac{4}{5} \div \frac{18}{25} = \frac{\overset{2}{\cancel{4}}}{\underset{1}{\cancel{5}}} \times \frac{\overset{5}{\cancel{25}}}{\underset{9}{\cancel{18}}} = \frac{10}{9} = \mathbf{1\frac{1}{9}}$

24. $\overset{20}{\cancel{80}} \times \frac{3}{\underset{1}{\cancel{4}}} = \mathbf{60\ calories}.$

25. $9\frac{1}{3} \times 60 = \frac{28}{\underset{1}{\cancel{3}}} \times \overset{20}{\cancel{60}} = \mathbf{560\ seconds}.$

26. $12 - 4 = 8$

    $\frac{8}{12} = \mathbf{\frac{2}{3}}$

    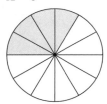

27. $\frac{20}{\frac{1}{2}} = 20 \times \frac{2}{1} = \mathbf{40\ doses}.$

    or $\frac{1\ dose}{\frac{1}{2}\ t} = \frac{X\ doses}{20\ t}$

    $\frac{1}{2}X = 20$

    $\frac{\frac{1}{2}X}{\frac{1}{2}} = \frac{20}{\frac{1}{2}}$

    $X = \frac{20}{1} \times \frac{2}{1}$

    $X = \mathbf{40\ doses}$

28. $3 \times 7 = 21$ doses.

    $21 \times 1\frac{1}{2} = 21 \times \frac{3}{2} = \frac{63}{2} = 2\overset{31\frac{1}{2}}{\overline{)63}} = \mathbf{31\frac{1}{2}}$
    $\quad\quad\quad\quad\quad\quad\quad\quad\quad\ \underline{-6}$
    $\quad\quad\quad\quad\quad\quad\quad\quad\quad\quad\ 3$
    $\quad\quad\quad\quad\quad\quad\quad\quad\quad\ \underline{-2}$
    $\quad\quad\quad\quad\quad\quad\quad\quad\quad\quad\ 1$

Review Set 4 (page 16)

1. **0.2; two-tenths**

2. $\frac{85}{100} = \mathbf{\frac{17}{20}};$ **0.85**

3. $1\frac{5}{100} = \mathbf{1\frac{1}{20}};$ **one and five-hundredths**

4. $\frac{6}{1000} = \mathbf{\frac{3}{500}};$ **six-thousandths**

5. **10.015; ten and fifteen-thousandths**
   $\quad 200\overset{0.015}{\overline{)3.000}}$
   $\quad\quad\ \underline{-2\ 00}$
   $\quad\quad\ \ \ 1\ 000$
   $\quad\quad\ \underline{-1\ 000}$
   $\quad\quad\quad\quad\ 0$

6. $\mathbf{1\frac{9}{10}};$ **one and nine-tenths**

7. $\mathbf{5\frac{1}{10}};$ **5.1**

8. **0.8; eight-tenths** $\quad \frac{4}{5} = 5\overset{0.8}{\overline{)4.0}}$
   $\quad\quad\quad\quad\quad\quad\quad\quad\ \underline{-4\ 0}$
   $\quad\quad\quad\quad\quad\quad\quad\quad\quad\ \ 0$

9. $250\frac{5}{10} = \mathbf{250\frac{1}{2}};$ **two hundred fifty and five-tenths**

10. **33.03; thirty-three and three-hundredths**

    $\quad 100\overset{0.03}{\overline{)3.00}}$
    $\quad\quad\ \underline{-3\ 00}$
    $\quad\quad\quad\quad\ 0$

11. $\frac{95}{100} = \mathbf{\frac{19}{20}};$ **ninety-five hundredths**

12. **2.75; two and seventy-five hundredths** $\quad 4\overset{0.75}{\overline{)3.00}}$
    $\quad\quad\quad\quad\quad\quad\quad\quad\quad\quad\quad\ \underline{-2\ 8}$
    $\quad\quad\quad\quad\quad\quad\quad\quad\quad\quad\quad\quad\ 20$
    $\quad\quad\quad\quad\quad\quad\quad\quad\quad\quad\ \underline{-20}$
    $\quad\quad\quad\quad\quad\quad\quad\quad\quad\quad\quad\quad\ 0$

13. $7\frac{5}{1000} = \mathbf{7\frac{1}{200}};$ **7.005** $\quad 200\overset{0.005}{\overline{)1.000}}$
    $\quad\quad\quad\quad\quad\quad\quad\quad\quad\quad\quad\ \underline{-1\ 000}$
    $\quad\quad\quad\quad\quad\quad\quad\quad\quad\quad\quad\quad\quad\ 0$

14. **0.084; eighty-four thousandths**

    $\frac{21}{250} = 250\overset{0.084}{\overline{)21.000}}$
    $\quad\quad\quad\ \underline{-20\ 00}$
    $\quad\quad\quad\quad\ 1\ 000$
    $\quad\quad\quad\ \underline{-1\ 000}$
    $\quad\quad\quad\quad\quad\ 0$

15. $12.125 = \frac{125}{1000} = 12\frac{1}{8}$;

    twelve and one hundred twenty-five thousandths

16. $20\frac{9}{100}$; **twenty and nine-hundredths**

17. $22\frac{22}{1000} = 22\frac{11}{500}$; **22.022**

$$\begin{array}{r} 0.022 \\ 1000\overline{)22.000} \\ -20\ 00 \\ \hline 2\ 000 \\ -2\ 000 \\ \hline 0 \end{array}$$

18. $0.15 = \frac{15}{100} = \frac{3}{20}$;

    fifteen-hundredths

19. **1000.005; one thousand and five-thousandths**

$$\begin{array}{r} 0.005 \\ 200\overline{)1.000} \end{array}$$

20. $4085\frac{75}{1000} = 4085\frac{3}{40}$;

    4085.075
$$\begin{array}{r} 0.075 \\ 40\overline{)3.000} \\ -2\ 80 \\ \hline 200 \\ -200 \\ \hline 0 \end{array}$$

Review Set 5 (page 18)

1. $\begin{array}{r} 0.160 \\ 5.375 \\ 1.050 \\ +16.000 \\ \hline \textbf{22.585} \end{array}$

2. $\begin{array}{r} 7.517 \\ 3.200 \\ 0.160 \\ +33.300 \\ \hline \textbf{44.177} \end{array}$

3. $\begin{array}{r} 13.009 \\ -0.700 \\ \hline \textbf{12.309} \end{array}$

4. $\begin{array}{r} 5.125 \\ 6.025 \\ +0.150 \\ \hline 11.300 = \textbf{11.30} \end{array}$

5. $\begin{array}{r} 175.100 \\ +0.099 \\ \hline \textbf{175.199} \end{array}$

6. $\begin{array}{r} 25.200 \\ +0.193 \\ \hline \textbf{25.007} \end{array}$

7. $\begin{array}{r} 0.580 \\ -0.062 \\ \hline \textbf{0.518} \end{array}$

8. $\begin{array}{r} \$10.10 \\ -0.62 \\ \hline \$\ \textbf{9.48} \end{array}$

9. $\begin{array}{r} \overset{8\ \ 9\,10}{\$19.\cancel{00}} \\ -0.09 \\ \hline \$\textbf{18.91} \end{array}$

10. $\begin{array}{r} \$\ 5.05 \\ 0.17 \\ +17.49 \\ \hline \$\textbf{22.71} \end{array}$

11. $\begin{array}{r} 4.000 \\ 1.980 \\ 0.420 \\ +0.003 \\ \hline \textbf{6.403} \end{array}$

12. $\begin{array}{r} 0.30 \\ -0.03 \\ \hline \textbf{0.27} \end{array}$

13. $\begin{array}{r} 16.30 \\ -12.15 \\ \hline \textbf{4.15} \end{array}$

14. $\begin{array}{r} 2.50 \\ -0.99 \\ \hline \textbf{1.51} \end{array}$

15. $\begin{array}{r} 5.00 \\ 2.50 \\ 0.05 \\ 0.15 \\ +2.55 \\ \hline \textbf{10.25} \end{array}$

16. $\begin{array}{r} 0.030 \\ 0.160 \\ +2.327 \\ \hline \textbf{2.517} \end{array}$

17. $\begin{array}{r} 700.00 \\ -325.65 \\ \hline \textbf{374.35} \end{array}$

18. $\begin{array}{r} 645.32 \\ -40.90 \\ \hline \textbf{604.42} \end{array}$

19. $\begin{array}{r} 18.000 \\ 2.350 \\ 7.006 \\ +0.093 \\ \hline \textbf{27.449} \end{array}$

20. $\begin{array}{r} 13.529 \\ +10.090 \\ \hline \textbf{23.619} \end{array}$

Review Set 6 (page 22)

1. $\begin{array}{r} 1.16 \\ \times\ 5.03 \\ \hline 348 \\ 000 \\ 580 \\ \hline 5.8348 = \textbf{5.83} \end{array}$

2. $\begin{array}{r} 0.314 \\ \times\ \ 7 \\ \hline 2.198 = \textbf{2.20} \end{array}$

3. $\begin{array}{r} 1.71 \\ \times\ 25 \\ \hline 855 \\ 342 \\ \hline \textbf{42.75} \end{array}$

4. $\begin{array}{r} 3.002 \\ \times\ \ 0.05 \\ \hline 0.15010 = \textbf{0.15} \end{array}$

5. $\begin{array}{r} 16.10 \\ \times\ 25.04 \\ \hline 6440 \\ 0000 \\ 8050 \\ 3220 \\ \hline 403.1440 = \textbf{403.14} \end{array}$

6. $\begin{array}{r} 75.10 \\ \times\ 1000.01 \\ \hline 7510 \\ 0000 \\ 0000 \\ 0000 \\ 0000 \\ 7510 \\ \hline 75100.7510 = \textbf{75,100.75} \end{array}$

7. $\begin{array}{r} 16.03 \\ \times\ \ 2.05 \\ \hline 8015 \\ 0000 \\ 3206 \\ \hline 32.8615 = \textbf{32.86} \end{array}$

8. $\begin{array}{r} 55.50 \\ \times\ \ 0.05 \\ \hline 2.7750 = \textbf{2.78} \end{array}$

9. $\begin{array}{r} 15.025 \\ \times\ \ 23.2 \\ \hline 30050 \\ 45075 \\ 30050 \\ \hline 348.5800 = \textbf{348.58} \end{array}$

10. $\begin{array}{r} 1.14 \\ \times\ 0.014 \\ \hline 456 \\ 114 \\ \hline 0.01596 = \textbf{0.02} \end{array}$

11. $16 \div 0.04 = \textbf{400}$

$\begin{array}{r} 4\ 00. \\ 0.04.\overline{)16.00.} \\ -16 \\ \hline 0\ 0 \end{array}$

12. $25.3 \div 6.76 = \textbf{3.74}$

$\begin{array}{r} 3.742 \\ 6.76.\overline{)25.30.000} \\ -20\ 28 \\ \hline 5\ 020 \\ -4\ 732 \\ \hline 2880 \\ -2704 \\ \hline 1760 \\ -1352 \\ \hline 408 \end{array}$

13. $0.02 \div 0.004 = \textbf{5}$

$\begin{array}{r} 5.0 \\ 0.004.\overline{)0.020.0} \\ -20 \\ \hline 0 \end{array}$

14. $45.5 \div 15.25 = \textbf{2.98}$

$\begin{array}{r} 2.983 \\ 15.25.\overline{)45.50.000} \\ -3050 \\ \hline 15000 \\ -13725 \\ \hline 12750 \\ -12200 \\ \hline 5500 \\ -4575 \\ \hline 925 \end{array}$

15. $515 \div 0.125 = \textbf{4120}$

$\begin{array}{r} 4\ 120 \\ .125.\overline{)515.000.} \\ -500 \\ \hline 150 \\ -125 \\ \hline 250 \\ -250 \\ \hline 00 \end{array}$

16. $73 \div 13.40 = \textbf{5.45}$

$\begin{array}{r} 5.447 \\ 13.40.\overline{)73.00.000} \\ -6700 \\ \hline 6000 \\ -5360 \\ \hline 6400 \\ -5360 \\ \hline 10400 \\ -9380 \\ \hline 1020 \end{array}$

17. $16.36 \div 0.06 = \textbf{272.67}$

$\begin{array}{r} 272.666 \\ 0.06.\overline{)16.36.000} \\ -12 \\ \hline 43 \\ -42 \\ \hline 16 \\ -12 \\ \hline 40 \\ -36 \\ \hline 40 \\ -36 \\ \hline 40 \\ -36 \\ \hline 4 \end{array}$

18. $0.375 \div 0.25 = \textbf{1.5}$

$\begin{array}{r} 1.5 \\ 0.25.\overline{)0.37.5} \\ -25 \\ \hline 125 \\ -125 \\ \hline 0 \end{array}$

19. $100.04 \div 0.002 = \textbf{50,020}$

$\begin{array}{r} 50\ 020 \\ .002.\overline{)100.040.} \\ -10 \\ \hline 0004 \\ -4 \\ \hline 00 \end{array}$

20. $45 \div 0.15 = \textbf{300}$

$\begin{array}{r} 3\ 00 \\ .15.\overline{)45.00.} \\ -45 \\ \hline 000 \end{array}$

21. $562.5 \times 100 = 562.50. = \textbf{56,250}$

22. $16 \times 10 = 16.0. = \textbf{160}$

23. $25 \div 1000 = .025. = \textbf{0.025}$

24. $32.005 \div 1000 = .032.005$
$= \textbf{0.032005}$

25. $0.125 \div 100 = .00.125 = \textbf{0.00125}$

26. $23.25 \times 10 = 23.2.5 = \textbf{232.5}$

27. $717.717 \div 10 = 71.7.717$
$= \textbf{71.7717}$

28. $83.16 \times 10 = 83.1.6 = \textbf{831.6}$

29. $0.33 \times 100 = 0.33. = \textbf{33}$

30. $14.106 \times 1000 = 14.106.$
$= \textbf{14,106}$

Review Set 7 (page 23)

1. **0.4;** $\frac{2}{5}$; **40%; 2:5**

   $\frac{2}{5} \times \frac{20}{20} = \frac{40}{100}$

2. 0.05; $\frac{5}{100} = \frac{1}{20}$; **5%; 1:20**

3. **0.17;** $\frac{17}{100}$; 17%; **17:100**

4. **0.25;** $\frac{1}{4}$; **25%; 1:4**

   $\frac{1}{4} \times \frac{25}{25} = \frac{25}{100}$

5. **0.06;** $\frac{6}{100} = \frac{3}{50}$; 6%; **3:50**

6. **0.17;** $\frac{1}{6}$; $16\frac{2}{3}$% or **17%; 1:6**

$$6)\overline{1.0}$$
$$\begin{array}{r} 0.166\ldots \\ 6)\overline{1.0} \\ -6 \\ \hline 40 \\ -36 \\ \hline 40 \\ -36 \\ \hline 40 \end{array}$$

7. **0.5;** $\frac{50}{100} = \frac{1}{2}$; 50%; **1:2**

8. **0.01;** $\frac{1}{100}$; **1%;** 1:100

9. 0.09; $\frac{9}{100}$; **9%; 9:100**

10. 0.375 or **0.38;** $\frac{3}{8}$; 37.5% or **38%; 3:8**

$$\begin{array}{r} 0.375 \\ 8)\overline{3.0} \\ -24 \\ \hline 60 \\ -56 \\ \hline 40 \\ -40 \\ \hline 0 \end{array}$$

11. **0.67;** $\frac{2}{3}$; $66\frac{2}{3}$% or **67%; 2:3**

$$\begin{array}{r} 0.666\ldots \\ 3)\overline{2.0} \\ -18 \\ \hline 20 \\ -18 \\ \hline 20 \\ -18 \\ \hline 20 \end{array}$$

12. **0.33;** $\frac{1}{3}$; $33\frac{1}{3}$% or **33%; 1:3**

$$\begin{array}{r} 0.333\ldots \\ 3)\overline{1.0} \\ -9 \\ \hline 10 \\ -9 \\ \hline 10 \end{array}$$

13. 0.52; $\frac{52}{100} = \frac{13}{25}$; 52%; **13:25**

14. **0.45;** $\frac{9}{20}$; **45%;** 9:20

   $\frac{9}{20} \times \frac{5}{5} = \frac{45}{100}$

15. **0.86;** $\frac{6}{7}$; **86%; 6:7**

$$\begin{array}{r} 0.857 \\ 7)\overline{6.0} \\ -56 \\ \hline 40 \\ -35 \\ \hline 50 \\ -49 \\ \hline 1 \end{array}$$

16. **0.3;** $\frac{3}{10}$; **30%;** 3:10

   $\frac{3}{10} \times \frac{10}{10} = \frac{30}{100}$

17. **0.02;** $\frac{1}{50}$; **2%; 1:50**

   $\frac{1}{50} \times \frac{2}{2} = \frac{2}{100}$

18. 0.6; $\frac{6}{10} = \frac{3}{5}$; **60%; 3:5**

19. 0.04; $\frac{4}{100} = \frac{1}{25}$; **4%; 1:25**

20. **0.1;** $\frac{10}{100} = \frac{1}{10}$; 10%; **1:10**

Review Set 8 (page 29)

1. $\frac{1000}{2} = \frac{125}{X}$

   $1000X = 250$

   $\frac{1000X}{1000} = \frac{250}{1000}$

   $X = \frac{1}{4} = \mathbf{0.25}$

2. $\frac{500}{1.8} = \frac{250}{X}$

   $500X = 450$

   $\frac{500X}{500} = \frac{450}{500}$

   $X = \frac{450}{500} = \frac{45}{50} = \frac{9}{10} = 0.9$

   $X = \mathbf{0.9}$

3. $\frac{500}{1} = \frac{280}{X}$

   $500X = 280$

   $\frac{500X}{500} = \frac{280}{500}$

   $X = \frac{280}{500} = \frac{28}{50} = \frac{14}{25}$

   $\frac{14}{25} \times \frac{4}{4} = \frac{56}{100} = 0.56$

   $X = \mathbf{0.56}$

4. $\frac{0.5}{2} = \frac{250}{X}$

   $0.5X = 500$

   $\frac{0.5X}{0.5} = \frac{500}{0.5}$

$$\begin{array}{r} 100\,0. \\ 0.5)\overline{500.0} \\ -5 \\ \hline 000 \end{array}$$

   $X = \mathbf{1000}$

5. $\dfrac{75}{1.5} = \dfrac{35}{X}$

$75X = 52.5$

$\dfrac{75X}{75} = \dfrac{52.5}{75}$

$X = \mathbf{0.7}$

$$\begin{array}{r} 35 \\ \times\,1.5 \\ \hline 175 \\ 35 \\ \hline 52.5 \end{array}$$

$$\begin{array}{r} 0.7 \\ 75\overline{)52.5} \\ -52.5 \\ \hline 0 \end{array}$$

6. $\dfrac{X}{12} = \dfrac{1200}{28}$

$28X = 14400$

$\dfrac{28X}{28} = \dfrac{14400}{28}$

$X = \mathbf{514.29}$

$$\begin{array}{r} 1200 \\ \times\,12 \\ \hline 2400 \\ 1200 \\ \hline 14400 \end{array}$$

$$\begin{array}{r} 514.285 \\ 28\overline{)14400} \\ -140 \\ \hline 40 \\ -28 \\ \hline 120 \\ -112 \\ \hline 80 \\ -56 \\ \hline 240 \\ -224 \\ \hline 160 \\ -140 \\ \hline 20 \end{array}$$

7. $\dfrac{X}{60} = \dfrac{1000}{28}$

$28X = 60,000$

$\dfrac{28X}{28} = \dfrac{60,000}{28}$

$X = \mathbf{2142.86}$

$$\begin{array}{r} 2142.857 \\ 28\overline{)60000.000} \\ -56 \\ \hline 40 \\ -28 \\ \hline 120 \\ -112 \\ \hline 80 \\ -56 \\ \hline 240 \\ -224 \\ \hline 160 \\ -140 \\ \hline 200 \\ -196 \\ \hline 4 \end{array}$$

8. $\dfrac{2000}{X} = \dfrac{2}{0.5}$

$2X = 1000$

$\dfrac{2X}{2} = \dfrac{1000}{2}$

$X = \mathbf{500}$

$$\begin{array}{r} 2000 \\ \times\,0.5 \\ \hline 1000.0 \end{array}$$

9. $\dfrac{500}{X} = \dfrac{15}{6}$

$15X = 3000$

$\dfrac{15X}{15} = \dfrac{3000}{15} = \dfrac{\overset{200}{\cancel{3000}}}{\underset{1}{\cancel{15}}} = 200$

$X = \mathbf{200}$

10. $\dfrac{\frac{1}{4}}{500} = \dfrac{\frac{2.5}{100}}{X}$

$\dfrac{1}{4}X = \dfrac{\cancel{500}}{1} \times \dfrac{2.5}{\cancel{100}}_{1}$

$\dfrac{1}{4}X = 12.5$

$\dfrac{\frac{1}{4}X}{\frac{1}{4}} = \dfrac{12.5}{\frac{1}{4}}$

$X = 12.5 \times \dfrac{4}{1} = 50$

$X = \mathbf{50}$

$$\begin{array}{r} 12.5 \\ \times\,4 \\ \hline 50.0 \end{array}$$

11. $\dfrac{250}{1} = \dfrac{750}{X}$

$250X = 750$

$\dfrac{250X}{250} = \dfrac{750}{250}$

$X = \mathbf{3}$

$$\begin{array}{r} 3 \\ 250\overline{)750} \\ -750 \\ \hline 0 \end{array}$$

12. $\dfrac{80}{5} = \dfrac{10}{X}$

$80X = 50$

$\dfrac{80X}{80} = \dfrac{5\cancel{0}}{8\cancel{0}}$

$X = \dfrac{5}{8}$

$X = 0.625 = \mathbf{0.63}$

$$\begin{array}{r} 0.625 \\ 8\overline{)5.0} \\ -48 \\ \hline 20 \\ -16 \\ \hline 40 \end{array}$$

13. $\dfrac{5}{20} = \dfrac{X}{40}$

$20X = 200$

$X = \dfrac{20\cancel{0}}{2\cancel{0}}$

$X = \dfrac{20}{2}$

$X = \mathbf{10}$

14. $\dfrac{\frac{1}{100}}{1} = \dfrac{\frac{1}{150}}{X}$

$\dfrac{1}{100}X = \dfrac{1}{150}$

$\dfrac{\frac{1}{100}X}{\frac{1}{100}} = \dfrac{\frac{1}{150}}{\frac{1}{100}}$

$X = \dfrac{\frac{1}{150}}{\frac{1}{100}}$

$X = \dfrac{1}{150} \times \dfrac{100}{1} = \dfrac{100}{150}$

$X = \dfrac{2}{3} = 0.666 = \mathbf{0.67}$

$$\begin{array}{r} 0.666\ldots \\ 3\overline{)2.000} \\ -18 \\ \hline 20 \\ -18 \\ \hline 20 \\ -18 \\ \hline 2 \end{array}$$

15. $\dfrac{2.2}{X} = \dfrac{8.8}{5}$

$8.8X = 11$

$\dfrac{8.8X}{8.8} = \dfrac{11}{8.8}$

$X = \mathbf{1.25}$

$$\begin{array}{r} 2.2 \\ 5 \\ \hline 11.0 \end{array}$$

$$\begin{array}{r} 1.25 \\ 8.8\overline{)11.0.00} \\ -88 \\ \hline 220 \\ -176 \\ \hline 440 \\ -440 \\ \hline 0 \end{array}$$

16. $\dfrac{125}{\overset{\cancel{60}}{4}} \times \dfrac{\overset{1}{\cancel{15}}}{1} = X$

$\dfrac{125}{4} = X$

$X = \mathbf{31.25}$

$$\begin{array}{r} 31.25 \\ 4\overline{)125.00} \\ -12 \\ \hline 05 \\ -4 \\ \hline 10 \\ -8 \\ \hline 20 \\ -20 \\ \hline 0 \end{array}$$

17. $\dfrac{100}{\cancel{60}} \times \dfrac{\cancel{10}}{1} = X$

$\dfrac{100}{6} = X$

$X = \mathbf{16.67}$

$$\begin{array}{r} 16.666 \\ 6\overline{)100.000} \\ -6 \\ \hline 40 \\ -36 \\ \hline 40 \\ -36 \\ \hline 40 \\ -36 \\ \hline 40 \\ -36 \\ \hline 4 \end{array}$$

18. $\dfrac{80}{X} \times \dfrac{60}{1} = 20$

$\dfrac{4800}{X} = \dfrac{20}{1}$

$20X = 4800$

$\dfrac{20X}{20} = \dfrac{4800}{20}$

$X = \dfrac{480\cancel{0}}{2\cancel{0}}$

$X = \mathbf{240}$

$$\begin{array}{r} 240 \\ 2\overline{)480} \\ -4 \\ \hline 08 \\ -8 \\ \hline 0 \end{array}$$

19. $\dfrac{6}{X} \times 0.5 = 4$

$\dfrac{3}{X} = \dfrac{4}{1}$

$4X = 3$

$\dfrac{4X}{4} = \dfrac{3}{4}$

$X = \dfrac{3}{4} = \mathbf{0.75}$

$$\begin{array}{r} 0.5 \\ \times\ 6 \\ \hline 3.0 \end{array} \qquad \begin{array}{r} 0.75 \\ 4\overline{)3.00} \\ -28 \\ \hline 20 \\ -20 \\ \hline 0 \end{array}$$

20. $\dfrac{X}{5} \times 2.2 = 1$

$\dfrac{2.2X}{5} = \dfrac{1}{1}$

$2.2X = 5$

$\dfrac{2.2X}{2.2} = \dfrac{5}{2.2}$

$X = \mathbf{2.27}$

$$\begin{array}{r} 2.272 \\ 2.2\overline{)5.0,000} \\ -4\,4 \\ \hline 60 \\ -44 \\ \hline 160 \\ -154 \\ \hline 60 \\ -44 \\ \hline 16 \end{array}$$

21. $\dfrac{X}{\frac{1}{4}} \times 15 = 60$

$\dfrac{15X}{\frac{1}{4}} = \dfrac{60}{1}$

$15X = \dfrac{1}{\cancel{4}} \times \overset{15}{\cancel{60}}$

$15X = 15$

$\dfrac{15X}{15} = \dfrac{15}{15}$

$X = \mathbf{1}$

22. $\dfrac{5}{25\%} \times 30\% = X$

$\dfrac{5X.3}{.25} = X$

$\dfrac{1.5}{0.25} = X$

$X = \mathbf{6}$

$30\% = \dfrac{30}{100} = \dfrac{3}{10} = 0.3$

$25\% = \dfrac{25}{100} = 0.25$

$$\begin{array}{r} 6. \\ 0.25\overline{)1.50.} \\ -150 \\ \hline \end{array}$$

Practice Problems—Chapter 1 (page 29)

1. 14 = **XIV**

2. 25 = **XXV**

3. 8 = **VIII**

4. 20 = **XX**

5. VII = **7**

6. XXIV = **24**

7. XIX = **19**

8. XXX = **30**

9. $\dfrac{1}{4} + \dfrac{2}{3} = \dfrac{3}{12} + \dfrac{8}{12} = \mathbf{\dfrac{11}{12}}$

10. $\dfrac{6}{7} - \dfrac{1}{9} = \dfrac{54}{63} - \dfrac{7}{63} = \mathbf{\dfrac{47}{63}}$

11. $1\dfrac{3}{5} \times \dfrac{5}{8} = \dfrac{8}{5} \times \dfrac{5}{8} = \dfrac{\overset{1}{\cancel{40}}}{\underset{1}{\cancel{40}}} = \mathbf{1}$

12. $\dfrac{3}{8} \div \dfrac{3}{4} = \dfrac{\overset{1}{\cancel{3}}}{\underset{2}{\cancel{8}}} \times \dfrac{\overset{1}{\cancel{4}}}{\underset{1}{\cancel{3}}} = \mathbf{\dfrac{1}{2}}$

13. $\begin{array}{r} 13.200 \\ 32.550 \\ +\ 0.029 \\ \hline 45.779 = \mathbf{45.78} \end{array}$

14. $\begin{array}{r} 80.30 \\ -21.06 \\ \hline 59.24 \end{array}$

15. $0.3 \times 0.3 = \mathbf{0.09}$

$\begin{array}{r} 0.3 \\ \times\ 0.3 \\ \hline 0.09 \end{array}$

16. $1.5 \div 0.125 = \textbf{12}$

$$0.125.\overline{)1.500.}$$
$$\underline{-125}$$
$$250$$
$$\underline{-250}$$
$$0$$

17. $\frac{1}{150} \div \frac{1}{100}$

$$\frac{1}{150} \times \frac{100}{1} = \frac{100}{150} = \frac{\overset{2}{\cancel{10}}}{\underset{3}{\cancel{15}}} = \frac{\textbf{2}}{\textbf{3}}$$

18. $\frac{\frac{1}{120}}{\frac{1}{60}} = \frac{1}{120} \times \frac{60}{1} = \frac{60}{120} = \frac{\overset{1}{\cancel{6}}}{\underset{2}{\cancel{12}}} = \frac{\textbf{1}}{\textbf{2}}$

19. $20\% \times 0.09 =$
$0.20 \times 0.09 = \textbf{0.02}$

$$0.20$$
$$\underline{\times 0.09}$$
$$0.0180 = 0.02$$

20. $\frac{16\%}{\frac{1}{4}} = 16\% \times \frac{4}{1} = 0.16 \times 4 = \textbf{0.64}$

$$0.16$$
$$\underline{\times 4}$$
$$0.64$$

21. $\frac{1}{3}$, $\frac{1}{2}$, $\frac{1}{6}$, $\frac{1}{10}$, $\frac{1}{5}$

0.33, 0.50, 0.17, 0.10, 0.20

    (4)   (5)   (2)   (1)   (3)

or, all have the same numerator; smallest fraction has the largest denominator

$\frac{\textbf{1}}{\textbf{10}}$, $\frac{\textbf{1}}{\textbf{6}}$, $\frac{\textbf{1}}{\textbf{5}}$, $\frac{\textbf{1}}{\textbf{3}}$, $\frac{\textbf{1}}{\textbf{2}}$
     (smallest to largest)

22. $\frac{3}{4}$, $\frac{7}{8}$, $\frac{5}{6}$, $\frac{2}{3}$, $\frac{9}{10}$

0.75, 0.88, 0.83, 0.67, 0.90

    (2)   (4)   (3)   (1)   (5)

$\frac{\textbf{2}}{\textbf{3}}$, $\frac{\textbf{3}}{\textbf{4}}$, $\frac{\textbf{5}}{\textbf{6}}$, $\frac{\textbf{7}}{\textbf{8}}$, $\frac{\textbf{9}}{\textbf{10}}$
     (smallest to largest)

23. 0.250, 0.125, 0.3, 0.009, 0.1909

    (4)   (2)   (5)   (1)   (3)

0.009,   0.125,   0.1909,   0.250,   0.3

    (smallest to largest)

24. 0.9%; $\frac{1}{2}\%$; 50%; 500%; 100%

0.009; 0.005; 0.5; 5; 1

    (2)   (1)   (3)   (5)   (4)

$\frac{\textbf{1}}{\textbf{2}}\textbf{\%}$,   **0.9\%,   50\%,   100\%,   500\%**

    (smallest to largest)

25. $1 : 100 = \frac{1}{100} = \textbf{0.01}$

26. $\frac{6}{150} = \textbf{0.04}$

$$150\overline{)6.00}$$
$$\underline{-600}$$
$$0$$

27. $0.009 = \frac{9 \div 10}{1000 \div 10} = \frac{0.9}{100} = \textbf{0.9\%}$

28. $33\frac{1}{3}\% = \frac{33\frac{1}{3}}{100} = \frac{\frac{100}{3}}{100} = \frac{\cancel{100}}{3} \times \frac{1}{\underset{1}{\cancel{100}}} = \frac{\textbf{1}}{\textbf{3}}$

29. $\frac{5}{9} = \textbf{5:9}$

30. $0.05 = \frac{5}{100} = \frac{\textbf{1}}{\textbf{20}}$

31. $\frac{1}{2}\% = 0.5\% = \frac{0.5}{100} = 0.5 \div 100 = 0.00.5 = 0.005$

$0.005 = \frac{5}{1000} = \frac{1}{200} = \textbf{1:200}$

32. $2 : 3 = \frac{\textbf{2}}{\textbf{3}}$

33. $3 : 4 = \frac{3}{4} = 0.75 = \textbf{75\%}$

$$0.75$$
$$4\overline{)3.0}$$
$$\underline{-28}$$
$$20$$
$$\underline{-20}$$
$$0$$

34. $\frac{2}{5} = 0.40 = \textbf{40\%}$

$$0.40$$
$$5\overline{)2.0}$$
$$\underline{-20}$$
$$0$$

35. $\frac{1}{6} = \textbf{0.17}$

$$0.166$$
$$6\overline{)1.0}$$
$$\underline{-6}$$
$$40$$
$$\underline{-36}$$
$$40$$
$$\underline{-36}$$
$$4$$

36. $\frac{0.35}{1.3} \times 4.5 = X$

$\frac{0.35}{1.3} \times \frac{4.5}{1} = X$

$\frac{1.575}{1.3} = X$

$X = \textbf{1.21}$

$$0.35$$
$$\underline{\times 4.5}$$
$$175$$
$$140$$
$$1.575$$

$$1.211$$
$$1.3.\overline{)1.5.75}$$
$$\underline{-13}$$
$$27$$
$$\underline{-26}$$
$$15$$
$$\underline{-13}$$
$$20$$

37. $\frac{0.3}{2.6} = \frac{0.15}{X}$

$0.3X = 0.39$

$\frac{0.3X}{0.3} = \frac{0.39}{0.3}$

$X = \textbf{1.3}$

$$0.15$$
$$\underline{2.6}$$
$$90$$
$$30$$
$$0.390$$

$$1.3$$
$$0.3.\overline{)0.3.9}$$
$$\underline{-3}$$
$$9$$
$$\underline{-9}$$
$$0$$

38. $\frac{1,500,000}{500,000} \times X = 7.5$

$\frac{\overset{3}{\cancel{15}}}{\underset{1}{\cancel{5}}} \times \frac{X}{1} = 7.5$

$3X = 7.5$

$\frac{3X}{3} = \frac{7.5}{3}$

$X = \textbf{2.5}$

$$\begin{array}{r} 2.5 \\ 3\overline{)7.5} \\ -6 \\ \hline 15 \\ -15 \\ \hline 0 \end{array}$$

39. $\frac{\frac{1}{4}}{1} = \frac{\frac{1}{6}}{X}$

$\frac{1}{4}X = \frac{1}{6}$

$\frac{\frac{1}{4}X}{\frac{1}{4}} = \frac{\frac{1}{6}}{\frac{1}{4}}$

$X = \frac{1}{6} \times \frac{4}{1} = \frac{2}{3}$

$X = \textbf{0.67}$

$$\begin{array}{r} 0.666 \\ 6\overline{)4.000} \\ -36 \\ \hline 40 \\ -36 \\ \hline 40 \end{array}$$

40. $\frac{1:4}{2500} = \frac{1:100}{X}$

$\frac{\frac{1}{4}}{2500} = \frac{\frac{1}{100}}{X}$

$\frac{1}{4}X = \frac{1}{\cancel{100}} \times \frac{\overset{25}{\cancel{2500}}}{1}$

$\frac{\frac{1}{4}X}{\frac{1}{4}} = \frac{25}{\frac{1}{4}}$

$X = 25 \times \frac{4}{1}$

$X = \textbf{100}$

41. $\frac{0.125}{2} = \frac{0.25}{X}$

$0.125X = 0.50$

$\frac{0.125X}{0.125} = \frac{0.50}{0.125}$

$X = \textbf{4}$

$$\begin{array}{r} 4 \\ 0.125\overline{)0.500.} \\ -500 \\ \hline 0 \end{array}$$

42. $\frac{\frac{1}{2}\%}{1000} = \frac{10\%}{X}$

$\frac{0.005}{1000} = \frac{0.1}{X}$

$0.005X = 100$

$\frac{0.005X}{0.005} = \frac{100}{0.005}$

$X = \textbf{20,000}$

$\frac{1}{2}\% = 0.5\% = 0.005$

$10\% = \frac{\cancel{10}}{\cancel{100}} = 0.1$

$$\begin{array}{r} 20,000 \\ 0.005\overline{)100.000} \\ -10 \\ \hline 00000 \end{array}$$

43. $\frac{\frac{1}{100}}{\frac{1}{150}} \times 2.2 = X$

$\frac{1}{\underset{2}{\cancel{100}}} \times \frac{\overset{3}{\cancel{150}}}{1} \times \frac{2.2}{1} = X$

$\frac{6.6}{2} = X$

$X = \textbf{3.3}$

$$\begin{array}{r} 3.3 \\ 2\overline{)6.6} \end{array}$$

44. $\frac{X}{15} = \frac{150}{7.5}$

$7.5X = 2250$

$\frac{75X}{75} = \frac{2250}{75}$

$X = \textbf{300}$

$$\begin{array}{r} 150 \\ \times 15 \\ \hline 750 \\ 150 \\ \hline 2250 \end{array}$$

$$\begin{array}{r} 300 \\ 7.5\overline{)2250.0} \\ -225 \\ \hline 00 \end{array}$$

45. $\frac{1,000,000}{600,000} \times 5 = X$

$\frac{10}{6} \times \frac{5}{1} = X$

$\frac{50}{6} = X$

$X = \textbf{8.33}$

$$\begin{array}{r} 8.333 \\ 6\overline{)50} \\ -48 \\ \hline 20 \\ -18 \\ \hline 20 \\ -18 \\ \hline 20 \end{array}$$

46. 1 nurse : 6 patients = X nurses : 30 patients

$\frac{1}{6} = \frac{X}{30}$

$6X = 30$

$\frac{6X}{6} = \frac{30}{6}$

$X = \textbf{5 nurses}$

47. 1 dime : \$0.10 = X dimes : \$1.10

$\frac{1}{\$0.10} = \frac{X}{\$1.10}$

$\$0.10X = \$1.10$

$\frac{\$0.10X}{\$0.10} = \frac{\$1.10}{\$0.10}$

$X = \textbf{11 dimes}$

$$\begin{array}{r} 11 \\ 0.10\overline{)1.10} \\ -10 \\ \hline 10 \\ -10 \\ \hline 0 \end{array}$$

48. $3\frac{1}{2}$ lb $\times$ \$0.69 = 3.5 $\times$ 0.69

$3.5 \times 0.69 = \$2.42$

$$\begin{array}{r} 3.5 \\ \times 0.69 \\ \hline 315 \\ 210 \\ \hline \$2.415 = \textbf{\$2.42} \end{array}$$

49. 3 water : 1 juice = X water : 4 juice

$\frac{3}{1} = \frac{X}{4}$

$X = \textbf{12}$

50. 1 cm : $\frac{3}{8}$ inch = X cm : 3 inches

$\frac{1}{\frac{3}{8}} = \frac{X}{3}$

$\frac{3}{8}X = 3$

$\frac{\frac{3}{8}X}{\frac{3}{8}} = \frac{3}{\frac{3}{8}}$

$X = \frac{3}{\frac{3}{8}}$

$X = 3 \times \frac{8}{3}$

$X = \frac{24}{3}$

$X = \textbf{8}$

Review Set 9 (page 33)

1. metric
2. volume
3. weight
4. length
5. $\frac{1}{1000}$ or **0.001**
6. **1000 mL**
7. **10 cc**
8. kilogram
9. milligram
10. **1000 cc**
11. **1 mg**
12. **2.2 lb**
13. **10 mm**
14. **0.3 g**
15. **1.33 mL**
16. **5 kg**
17. **1.5 mm**
18. **10 mg**
19. microgram
20. milliliter
21. cubic centimeter
22. gram
23. millimeter
24. kilogram
25. centimeter

Review Set 10 (page 36)

1. dram
2. ounce
3. minim
4. one-half
5. grain
6. ℥ ss
7. gr $\frac{1}{6}$

8. ℥ iv
9. pt ii
10. qt i $\frac{1}{4}$
11. gr x
12. ʒ viiiss
13. gr ii
14. pt 16
15. gr iii
16. ℥ 32
17. gr viss
18. 32
19. pt i
20. pt ii

Review Set 11 (page 37)

1. twenty drops
2. one thousand units
3. ten milliequivalents
4. four teaspoons
5. ten tablespoons
6. **4 gtt**
7. **30 mEq**
8. **5 T**
9. **1500 U**
10. **10 t**
11. False
12. units; U
13. **3 t**
14. **9 t**
15. **1000 mU**

Practice Problems—Chapter 2 (page 39)

1. milli
2. micro
3. centi

4. kilo
5. meter
6. gram
7. liter
8. drop
9. ounce
10. minim
11. grain
12. milligram
13. microgram
14. unit
15. milliequivalent
16. teaspoon
17. dram
18. milliliter
19. cubic centimeter
20. pint
21. tablespoon
22. millimeter
23. gram
24. centimeter
25. liter
26. meter
27. kilogram
28. gr ss
29. **2 t**
30. ℥ $\frac{1}{3}$
31. **500 mU**
32. **0.5 L**
33. gr $\frac{1}{4}$
34. gr $\frac{1}{200}$
35. **0.05 mg**

Review Set 12 (page 46)

1. 500 cc = **0.5 L**

$$\frac{1\text{ L}}{1000\text{ cc}} = \frac{X\text{ L}}{500\text{ cc}}$$

$$1000X = 500$$

$$\frac{1000X}{1000} = \frac{500}{1000}$$

$$X = \frac{1}{2} = 0.5\text{ L}$$

2. 0.015 g = **15 mg**

$$\frac{1\text{ g}}{1000\text{ mg}} = \frac{0.015\text{ g}}{X\text{ mg}}$$

$$X = 0.015 \times 1000$$

$$X = 15\text{ mg}$$

3. 8 mg = **0.008 g**

$$\frac{1\text{ g}}{1000\text{ mg}} = \frac{X\text{ g}}{8\text{ mg}}$$

$$1000X = 8$$

$$\frac{1000X}{1000} = \frac{8}{1000}$$

$$X = 0.008\text{ g}$$

4. 10 mg = **0.01 g**

$$\frac{1\text{ g}}{1000\text{ mg}} = \frac{X\text{ g}}{10\text{ mg}}$$

$$1000X = 10$$

$$\frac{1000X}{1000} = \frac{1\cancel{0}}{100\cancel{0}}$$

$$X = 0.01\text{ g}$$

5. 60 mg = **0.06 g**

$$\frac{1\text{ g}}{1000\text{ mg}} = \frac{X\text{ g}}{60\text{ mg}}$$

$$1000X = 60$$

$$\frac{1000X}{1000} = \frac{6\cancel{0}}{100\cancel{0}}$$

$$X = 0.06\text{ g}$$

6. 300 mg = **0.3 g**

$$\frac{1\text{ g}}{1000\text{ mg}} = \frac{X\text{ g}}{300\text{ mg}}$$

$$1000X = 300$$

$$\frac{1000X}{1000} = \frac{3\cancel{00}}{10\cancel{00}}$$

$$X = 0.3\text{ g}$$

7. 0.2 mg = **0.0002 g**

$$\frac{1\text{ g}}{1000\text{ mg}} = \frac{X\text{ g}}{0.2\text{ mg}}$$

$$1000X = 0.2$$

$$\frac{1000X}{1000} = \frac{0.2}{1000}$$

$$X = 0.000.2 \div 1000$$

$$X = 0.0002\text{ g}$$

8. 1.2 g = **1200 mg**

$$\frac{1\text{ g}}{1000\text{ mg}} = \frac{1.2\text{ g}}{X\text{ mg}}$$

$$X = 1.2 \times 1000$$

$$X = 1.200 \times 1000$$

$$X = 1200\text{ mg}$$

9. 0.0025 kg = **2.5 g**

$$\frac{1\text{ kg}}{1000\text{ g}} = \frac{0.0025\text{ kg}}{X\text{ g}}$$

$$X = 0.0025 \times 1000$$

$$X = 2.5\text{ g}$$

10. 0.065 g = **65 mg**

$$\frac{1\text{ g}}{1000\text{ mg}} = \frac{0.065\text{ g}}{X\text{ mg}}$$

$$X = 0.065 \times 1000$$

$$X = 65\text{ mg}$$

11. 0.005 L = **5 mL**

$$\frac{1\text{ L}}{1000\text{ mL}} = \frac{0.005\text{ L}}{X\text{ mL}}$$

$$X = 0.005 \times 1000$$

$$X = 5\text{ mL}$$

12. 1.5 L = **1500 cc**

$$\frac{1\text{ L}}{1000\text{ cc}} = \frac{1.5\text{ L}}{X\text{ cc}}$$

$$X = 1.5 \times 1000$$

$$= 1.500 \times 1000$$

$$X = 1500\text{ cc}$$

13. 2 mL = **2 cc**

1 mL = 1 cc, 2 mL = 2 cc

14. 250 cc = **0.25 L**

$$\frac{1\text{ L}}{1000\text{ cc}} = \frac{X\text{ L}}{250\text{ cc}}$$

$$1000X = 250$$

$$\frac{1000X}{1000} = \frac{250}{1000}$$

$$X = \frac{\overset{1}{\cancel{250}}}{\underset{4}{\cancel{1000}}}$$

$$X = \frac{1}{4} = 0.25\text{ L}$$

15. 2 kg = **2000 g**

$$\frac{1\text{ kg}}{1000\text{ g}} = \frac{2\text{ kg}}{X\text{ g}}$$

$$X = 2 \times 1000$$

$$X = 2000\text{ g}$$

16. 56.08 cc = **56.08 mL**

1 cc = 1 mL

56.08 cc = 56.08 mL

17. 79,200 mL = **79.2 L**

$$\frac{1\,L}{1000\,mL} = \frac{X\,L}{79,200\,mL}$$
$$1000X = 79,200$$
$$\frac{1000X}{1000} = \frac{79,200}{1000}$$
$$X = 79.200 \div 1000$$
$$X = 79.2\,L$$

18. 1 L = **1000 mL**

19. 1 g = **1000 mg**

20. 1 mL = **0.001 L**

$$\frac{1\,L}{1000\,mL} = \frac{X\,L}{1\,mL}$$
$$1000X = 1$$
$$\frac{1000X}{1000} = \frac{1}{1000}$$
$$X = 0.001\,L$$

21. 0.23 mcg = **0.00023 mg**

$$\frac{1\,mg}{1000\,mcg} = \frac{X\,mg}{0.23\,mcg}$$
$$1000X = 0.23$$
$$\frac{1000X}{1000} = \frac{0.23}{1000}$$
$$X = 0.23 \div 1000$$
$$X = 0000.23 \div 1000$$
$$X = 0.00023\,mg$$

22. 1.05 g = **0.00105 kg**

$$\frac{1\,kg}{1000\,g} = \frac{X\,kg}{1.05\,g}$$
$$1000X = 1.05$$
$$\frac{1000X}{1000} = \frac{1.05}{1000}$$
$$X = 1.05 \div 1000$$
$$X = 0001.05 \div 1000$$
$$X = 0.00105\,kg$$

23. 0.01 mcg = **0.00001 mg**

$$\frac{1\,mg}{1000\,mcg} = \frac{X\,mg}{0.01\,mcg}$$
$$\frac{1000X}{1000} = \frac{0.01}{1000}$$
$$X = 0.01 \div 1000$$
$$X = 0000.01 \div 1000$$
$$X = 0.00001\,mg$$

24. 0.4 mg = **400 mcg**

$$\frac{1\,mg}{1000\,mcg} = \frac{0.4\,mg}{X\,mcg}$$
$$X = 0.4 \times 1000$$
$$X = 0.400 \times 1000$$
$$X = 400\,mcg$$

25. 25 g = **0.025 kg**

$$\frac{1\,kg}{1000\,g} = \frac{X\,kg}{25\,g}$$
$$1000X = 25$$
$$\frac{1000X}{1000} = \frac{25}{1000}$$
$$X = 0.025$$

26. 50 cm = **0.5 m**

$$\frac{1\,m}{100\,cm} = \frac{X\,m}{50\,cm}$$
$$100X = 50$$
$$\frac{100X}{100} = \frac{50}{100}$$
$$X = 0.5\,m$$

27. 10 L = **10,000 mL**

$$\frac{1\,L}{1000\,mL} = \frac{10\,L}{X\,mL}$$
$$X = 10,000\,mL$$

28. 450 cc = **0.45 L**

$$\frac{1\,L}{1000\,cc} = \frac{X\,L}{450\,cc}$$
$$1000X = 450$$
$$\frac{1000X}{1000} = \frac{450}{1000}$$
$$X = 0.45\,L$$

29. 5 mL = **0.005 L**

$$\frac{1\,L}{1000\,mL} = \frac{X\,L}{5\,mL}$$
$$1000X = 5$$
$$\frac{1000X}{1000} = \frac{5}{1000}$$
$$X = 0.005\,L$$

30. 30 mg = **30,000 mcg**

$$\frac{1\,mg}{1000\,mcg} = \frac{30\,mg}{X\,mcg}$$
$$X = 30,000\,mcg$$

Review Set 13 (page 49)

1. gr ss **= 30 mg**   **gr i = 60 mg**

$$\frac{\text{gr i}}{60 \text{ mg}} = \frac{\text{gr ss}}{\text{X mg}}$$

$$X = \frac{1}{2} \times 60$$

$$X = 30 \text{ mg}$$

2. gr $\frac{3}{4}$ **= 45 mg**   **gr i = 60 mg**

$$\frac{\text{gr i}}{60 \text{ mg}} = \frac{\text{gr}\frac{3}{4}}{\text{X mg}}$$

$$X = \frac{3}{\cancel{4}} \times \overset{15}{\cancel{60}}$$

$$1$$

$$X = 45 \text{ mg}$$

3. 0.03 g **= gr $\frac{9}{20}$**   **1 g = gr 15**

$$\frac{1 \text{ g}}{\text{gr 15}} = \frac{0.03 \text{ g}}{\text{gr X}}$$

$$X = 0.45 = \frac{45}{100} = \frac{9}{20}$$

$$X = \text{gr} \ \frac{9}{20}$$

4. gr $\frac{1}{150}$ **= 0.4 mg**   **gr i = 60 mg**

$$\frac{\text{gr i}}{60 \text{ mg}} = \frac{\text{gr}\frac{1}{150}}{\text{X mg}}$$

$$X = \frac{\cancel{60}}{1} \times \frac{1}{\cancel{150}} = \frac{6}{15} = \frac{2}{5}$$

$$X = 0.4 \text{ mg} \qquad 5\overline{)2.0}^{\ 0.4}$$

5. gr viiss **= 0.5 g**   **1 g = gr 15**

$$\frac{1 \text{ g}}{\text{gr 15}} = \frac{\text{X g}}{\text{gr viiss}}$$

$$\frac{1}{15} = \frac{X}{7.5}$$

$$15X = 7.5$$

$$\frac{15X}{15} = \frac{7.5}{15} \qquad 15\overline{)7.5}^{\ 0.5}$$

$$\qquad\qquad -75$$

$$X = 0.5 \text{ g} \qquad\quad \overline{0}$$

6. 15 mg **= gr $\frac{1}{4}$**   **gr i = 60 mg**

$$\frac{\text{gr i}}{60 \text{ mg}} = \frac{\text{gr X}}{15 \text{ mg}}$$

$$60X = 15$$

$$\frac{60X}{60} = \frac{15}{60}$$

$$X = \frac{1}{4}$$

$$X = \text{gr}\frac{1}{4}$$

7. 5 t **= 25 cc**   **1 t = 5 cc**

$$\frac{1 \text{ t}}{5 \text{ cc}} = \frac{5 \text{ t}}{\text{X cc}}$$

$$X = 25 \text{ cc}$$

8. 15 cc **= ℥ ss**   **℥ i = 30 cc**

$$\frac{℥ \text{ i}}{30 \text{ cc}} = \frac{℥ \text{ X}}{15 \text{ cc}}$$

$$30X = 15$$

$$\frac{30X}{30} = \frac{15}{30}$$

$$X = \frac{1}{2}$$

$$X = ℥\text{ss}$$

9. ℥ iiss = **75 mL**   ℥ i = 30 mL $\frac{℥\,i}{30\,mL} = \frac{℥\,iiss}{X\,mL}$ $\begin{array}{r} 30 \\ \times 2.5 \\ \hline 150 \\ 60 \\ \hline 75.0 \end{array}$

$$\frac{1}{30} = \frac{2.5}{X}$$
$$X = 2.5 \times 30$$
$$X = 75\ mL$$

10. 750 mL = **pt iss**   pt i = 500 mL $\frac{pt\,i}{500\,mL} = \frac{pt\,X}{750\,mL}$

$$500X = 750$$
$$\frac{500X}{500} = \frac{750}{500}$$
$$X = \frac{75\emptyset}{50\emptyset} = \frac{3}{2} = 1\frac{1}{2}$$
$$X = pt\ iss$$

11. 60 mL = **12 t**   1 t = 5 mL $\frac{1\,t}{5\,mL} = \frac{X\,t}{60\,mL}$

$$5X = 60$$
$$\frac{5X}{5} = \frac{60}{5}$$
$$X = 12\ t$$

12. 4 T = **60 cc**   1 T = 15 cc $\frac{1\,T}{15\,cc} = \frac{4\,T}{X\,cc}$

$$X = 60\ cc$$

13. 9 kg = **19.8 lb**   1 kg = 2.2 lb $\frac{1\,kg}{2.2\,lb} = \frac{9\,kg}{X\,lb}$ $\begin{array}{r} 2.2 \\ \times 9 \\ \hline 19.8 \end{array}$

$$X = 19.8\ lb$$

14. 110 lb. = **50 kg**   1 kg = 2.2 lb $\frac{1\,kg}{2.2\,lb} = \frac{X\,kg}{110\,lb}$

$$2.2X = 110$$
$$\frac{2.2X}{2.2} = \frac{110}{2.2}$$
$$X = 50\ kg$$

$$2.2\overline{)1100} \quad \begin{array}{r} 50. \\ -110 \\ \hline 00 \end{array}$$

15. 3 L = **℥ 96**   1 L = ℥ 32 $\frac{1\,L}{℥\,32} = \frac{3\,L}{℥\,X}$

$$X = 96$$
$$X = ℥\ 96$$

16. 3.5 kg = **7.7 lb**   1 kg = 2.2 lb $\frac{1\,kg}{2.2\,lb} = \frac{3.5\,kg}{X\,lb}$ $\begin{array}{r} 3.5 \\ \times 2.2 \\ \hline 70 \\ 70 \\ \hline 7.70 \end{array}$

$$X = 7.7\ lb$$

17. 12 in = **30 cm**   1 in = 2.5 cm $\frac{1\,in}{2.5\,cm} = \frac{12\,in}{X\,cm}$ $\begin{array}{r} 12 \\ \times 2.5 \\ \hline 60 \\ 24 \\ \hline 30.0 \end{array}$

$$X = 30\ cm$$

18. qt ii = **2 L**   qt i = 1 L

19. 3 t = **15 mL**   1 t = 5 mL $\frac{1\,t}{5\,mL} = \frac{3\,t}{X\,mL}$

$$X = 15\ mL$$

20. 99 lb = **45 kg**   **1 kg = 2.2 lb**

$$\frac{1\ kg}{2.2\ lb} = \frac{X\ kg}{99\ lb}$$

$$2.2X = 99$$

$$\frac{2.2X}{2.2} = \frac{99}{2.2}$$

$$X = 45\ kg$$

$$2.2\overline{)99.0} = 45.$$
$$-88$$
$$\overline{110}$$
$$-110$$
$$\overline{0}$$

21. 0.4 mg = **gr $\frac{1}{150}$**   **gr i = 60 mg**

$$\frac{gr\ i}{60\ mg} = \frac{gr\ X}{0.4\ mg}$$

$$60X = 0.4$$

$$\frac{60X}{60} = \frac{0.4}{60}$$

$$X = \frac{4}{10} \div \frac{60}{1}$$

$$X = \frac{\overset{1}{\cancel{4}}}{10} \times \frac{1}{\underset{15}{\cancel{60}}}$$

$$X = \frac{1}{150}$$

$$X = gr\ \frac{1}{150}$$

22. 0.6 mg = **gr $\frac{1}{100}$**   **gr i = 60 mg**

$$\frac{gr\ i}{60\ mg} = \frac{gr\ X}{0.6\ mg}$$

$$60X = 0.6$$

$$\frac{60X}{60} = \frac{0.6}{60}$$

$$X = \frac{6}{10} \div \frac{60}{1}$$

$$X = \frac{\overset{1}{\cancel{6}}}{10} \times \frac{1}{\underset{10}{\cancel{60}}}$$

$$X = \frac{1}{100}$$

$$X = gr\ \frac{1}{100}$$

23. pt i = **500 mL**   **pt i = 500 mL**

24. gr X = **600 mg**   **gr i = 60 mg**

$$\frac{gr\ i}{60\ mg} = \frac{gr\ x}{X\ mg}$$

$$\frac{1}{60} = \frac{10}{X}$$

$$X = 600\ mg$$

25. 300 mg = **gr v**   **gr i = 60 mg**

$$\frac{gr\ i}{60\ mg} = \frac{gr\ X}{300\ mg}$$

$$\frac{1}{60} = \frac{X}{300}$$

$$60X = 300$$

$$\frac{60X}{60} = \frac{300}{60}$$

$$X = \frac{300}{60} = 5$$

$$X = gr\ v$$

26. 30 cm = **12 in**   **1 in = 2.5 cm**

$$\frac{1\ in}{2.5\ cm} = \frac{X\ in}{30\ cm}$$

$$2.5X = 30$$

$$\frac{2.5X}{2.5} = \frac{30}{2.5}$$

$$X = 12\ in$$

$$2.5\overline{)30.0} = 12.$$
$$-25$$
$$\overline{50}$$
$$-50$$
$$\overline{0}$$

27. 90 mg = **gr iss**   **gr i = 60 mg**
$$\frac{\text{gr i}}{60 \text{ mg}} = \frac{\text{gr X}}{90 \text{ mg}}$$
$$\frac{1}{60} = \frac{X}{90}$$
$$60X = 90$$
$$\frac{60X}{60} = \frac{90}{60}$$
$$X = \frac{90}{60} = \frac{3}{2} = 1\frac{1}{2}$$
$$X = \text{gr iss}$$

28. 60 mL = **ʒ ii**   **ʒ i = 30 mL**
$$\frac{ʒ \text{ i}}{30 \text{ mL}} = \frac{ʒ \text{ X}}{60 \text{ mL}}$$
$$\frac{1}{30} = \frac{X}{60}$$
$$30X = 60$$
$$\frac{30X}{30} = \frac{60}{30}$$
$$X = 2$$
$$X = ʒ \text{ ii}$$

29. gr $\frac{1}{6}$ = **10 mg**   **gr i = 60 mg**
$$\frac{\text{gr i}}{60 \text{ mg}} = \frac{\text{gr}\frac{1}{6}}{X \text{ mg}}$$
$$X = \frac{1}{6} \times 60$$
$$X = 10 \text{ mg}$$

30. 30 mg = **gr ss**   **gr i = 60 mg**
$$\frac{\text{gr i}}{60 \text{ mg}} = \frac{\text{gr X}}{30 \text{ mg}}$$
$$\frac{1}{60} = \frac{X}{30}$$
$$60X = 30$$
$$\frac{60X}{60} = \frac{30}{60}$$
$$X = \frac{1}{2}$$
$$X = \text{gr ss}$$

31.   8 ounces milk
       6 ounces orange juice
       4 ounces water
       8 ounces iced tea
      10 ounces coffee
       4 ounces gelatin
       8 ounces water
       6 ounces tomato juice
       6 ounces beef broth
       5 ounces pudding
      12 ounces diet soda
       4 ounces water

       81 ounces total

$$\frac{ʒ \text{ i}}{30 \text{ mL}} = \frac{ʒ \text{ 81}}{X \text{ mL}}$$

$$X = \textbf{2430 mL}$$

$$\begin{array}{r} 81 \\ \times\, 30 \\ \hline 2430 \end{array}$$

32. $\dfrac{1 \text{ kg}}{2.2 \text{ lb}} = \dfrac{X \text{ kg}}{55 \text{ lb}}$

$2.2X = 55$

$\dfrac{2.2X}{2.2} = \dfrac{55}{2.2}$

$X = 25 \text{ kg}$

$\dfrac{0.05 \text{ mg}}{1 \text{ kg}} = \dfrac{X \text{ mg}}{25 \text{ kg}}$

$X = 1.25 \text{ mg}$

$$\begin{array}{r} 2\,5 \\ 2.2\overline{)55.0} \\ -44 \\ \hline 110 \\ -110 \\ \hline 0 \end{array}$$

$$\begin{array}{r} 25 \\ \times 0.05 \\ \hline 1.25 \end{array}$$

33. $\dfrac{1 \text{ T}}{15 \text{ mL}} = \dfrac{X \text{ T}}{60 \text{ mL}}$

$15X = 60$

$\dfrac{15X}{15} = \dfrac{60}{15}$

$X = 4 \text{ T}$

$1000 \text{ mL} = 1 \text{ L} = \text{qt i}$

Dissolve 4 tablespoons or 2 ounces Epsom Salts in 1 quart of water.

34. $\dfrac{1 \text{ t}}{5 \text{ mL}} = \dfrac{X \text{ t}}{10 \text{ mL}}$

$5X = 10$

$\dfrac{5X}{5} = \dfrac{10}{5}$

$X = 2 \text{ t}$

35. qt i = 32 ounces

infant is given 8 feedings of 4 ounces per day = 32 ounces/day

3 day supply = 3 quarts of formula.

Review Set 14 (page 52)

		EQUIVALENT

1. 0.5 mL = **0.0005 L**   **1000 mL = 1 L**   mL → L or smaller → larger; divide

0.5 mL = 0.5 ÷ 1000 = 0000.5 ÷ 1000 = 0.0005 L

2. 3 g = **gr 45**   **1 g = gr 15**   g → gr or larger → smaller; multiply

3 g = 3 × 15 = gr 45

3. 84 lb = **38.2 kg**   **2.2 lb = 1 kg**   lb → kg smaller → larger; divide

84 lb = 84 ÷ 2.2 = 38.2 kg

$$\begin{array}{r} 38.18 \\ 2.2\overline{)84.000} \\ -66 \\ \hline 180 \\ -176 \\ \hline 40 \\ -22 \\ \hline 180 \\ -176 \\ \hline 4 \end{array}$$

EQUIVALENT

4. gr xx = **1.3 g**   **15 gr = 1 g**

gr → g smaller → larger; divide

gr xx = 20 ÷ 15 = 1.3 g

$$\begin{array}{r} 1.33 \\ 15\overline{)20.00} \\ -15 \\ \hline 50 \\ -45 \\ \hline 50 \\ -45 \\ \hline 5 \end{array}$$

5. gr $\frac{1}{8}$ = **7.5 mg**   **gr i = 60 mg**

gr → mg larger → smaller; multiply

gr $\frac{1}{8} = \frac{1}{\overset{}{\underset{2}{8}}} \times \frac{\overset{15}{\cancel{60}}}{1} = \frac{15}{2} = 7.5$ mg

6. 75 mL = ℥ **iiss**   **30 mL = ℥ i**

mL → ℥ smaller → larger; divide

75 mL = 75 ÷ 30 = ℥ iiss

$$\begin{array}{r} 2.5 \\ 30\overline{)75.0} \\ -60 \\ \hline 150 \\ -150 \\ \hline 0 \end{array}$$

7. 750 mL = **pt iss**   **pt i = 500 mL**

mL → pt smaller → larger; divide

750 mL = 750 ÷ 500 = $\frac{75\cancel{0}}{50\cancel{0}} = \frac{3}{2} = 1\frac{1}{2}$ = pt iss

8. ℥ iss = **45 mL**   **℥ i = 30 mL**

℥ → mL larger → smaller; multiply

℥ iss = $1\frac{1}{2} \times 30 = \frac{3}{\underset{1}{2}} \times \overset{15}{\cancel{30}} = 45$ mL

9. 15 mg = **gr $\frac{1}{4}$**   **60 mg = gr i**

mg → gr smaller → larger; divide

15 mg = 15 ÷ 60 = $\frac{15}{60} = \frac{1}{4}$ = gr $\frac{1}{4}$

10. 0.625 mcg = **0.000625 mg**   **1000 mcg = 1 mg**

mcg → mg smaller → larger; divide

0.625 mcg = 0.625 ÷ 1000 = 0000.625 = 0.000625 mg

11. 2.5 mL = $\frac{1}{2}$ **t**   **5 mL = 1 t**

mL → t smaller → larger; divide

2.5 mL = 2.5 ÷ 5 = $\frac{1}{2}$ t

$$\begin{array}{r} 0.5 \\ 5\overline{)2.5} \\ -25 \\ \hline 0 \end{array} \qquad 0.5 = \frac{5}{10} = \frac{1}{2}$$

12. gr ss = **30 mg**   **gr i = 60 mg**

gr → mg larger → smaller; multiply

gr ss = $\frac{1}{2} \times 60 = 30$ mg

EQUIVALENT

13. 7.5 mg = **gr $\frac{1}{8}$**　　　　　**60 mg = gr i**　　　　mg → gr smaller → larger; divide

$$7.5 \text{ mg} = 7\frac{1}{2} \div 60 = \frac{\overset{1}{\cancel{15}}}{2} \times \frac{1}{\underset{4}{\cancel{60}}} = \frac{1}{8} = \text{gr } \frac{1}{8}$$

14. 0.6 mg = **gr $\frac{1}{100}$**　　　　**60 mg = gr i**　　　mg → gr smaller → larger; divide

$$0.6 \text{ mg} = \frac{6}{10} \div 60 = \frac{\overset{1}{\cancel{6}}}{10} \times \frac{1}{\underset{10}{\cancel{60}}} = \frac{1}{100} = \text{gr } \frac{1}{100}$$

15. 7.5 cm = **3 in**　　　　　　**2.5 cm = 1 in**　　　cm → in smaller → larger; divide

$$7.5 \text{ cm} = 7.5 \div 2.5 = 3 \text{ in} \qquad 2.5\overline{)7.5} \\ \underline{-75} \\ 0$$

16. 16 g = **16,000 mg**　　　　**1 g = 1000 mg**　　　g → mg larger → smaller; multiply
16 g = 16 × 1000 = 16,000 mg

17. 15 mL = **ʒ ss**　　　　　　**ʒ i = 30 mL**　　　mL → ʒ smaller → larger; divide
15 mL = 15 ÷ 30 = $\frac{1}{2}$ = ʒ ss

18. **ʒ 16 = qt ss**　　　　　　**ʒ 32 = qt i**　　　ʒ → qt smaller → larger; divide
ʒ 16 = 16 ÷ 32 = $\frac{1}{2}$ = qt ss

19. qt ii = **2 L**　　　　　　　**qt i = 1 L**　　　qt → L same relative size; qt i = 1 L
qt ii = 2 L

20. pt i = **qt ss**　　　　　　　**pt ii = qt i**　　　pt → qt smaller → larger; divide
pt i = 1 ÷ 2 = $\frac{1}{2}$ = qt ss

21. 150 mL = **ʒ V**　　　　　　**30 mL = ʒ i**　　　mL → ʒ smaller → larger; divide
150 mL = 150 ÷ 30 = 5 ounces of juice = ʒ v

22. 5 mL = **1 t**　　　　　　　**5 mL = 1 t**　　　Give the child 1 teaspoon of Tylenol.

23. 2000 mL = **8 glasses**　　**2000 mL = 2 L = 2 quarts**　　The patient should have at least 8 8-ounce glasses
1 quart = 4 - 8 ounce cups　　of water each day.
2 quarts = 8 - 8 ounce cups

24. 50 lb = **22.7 kg**　　　　**2.2 lb = 1 kg**　　　lb → kg smaller → larger; divide
50 lb = 50 ÷ 2.2 = 22.7 kg

$$2.2\overline{)500} \\ \underline{-44} \\ 60 \\ \underline{-44} \\ 160 \\ \underline{-154} \\ 60 \\ \underline{-44} \\ 16$$

(quotient 22.72)

25. gr $\frac{1}{4}$ = **15 mg**　　　　**gr i = 60 mg**　　　gr → mg larger → smaller; multiply

$$\text{gr } \frac{1}{4} = \frac{1}{\underset{1}{\cancel{4}}} \times \overset{15}{\cancel{60}} = 15 \text{ mg}$$

Review Set 15 (page 55)

1. 0032 = **12:32 AM**

2. 0730 = **7:30 AM**

3. 1640 = 1640 − 1200 = **4:40 PM**

4. 2121 = 2121 − 1200 = **9:21 PM**

5. 2359 = 2359 − 1200 = **11:59 PM**

6. 1215 = **12:15 PM**

7. 0220 = **2:20 AM**

8. 1010 = **10:10 AM**

9. 1315 = 1315 − 1200 = **1:15 PM**

10. 1825 = 1825 − 1200 = **6:25 PM**

11. 1:30 PM = 1:30 + 12:00 = **1330**

12. 12:04 AM = **0004**

13. 9:45 PM = 9:45 + 12:00 = **2145**

14. 12:00 noon = **1200**

15. 11:15 PM = 11:15 + 12:00 = **2315**

16. 3:45 AM = **0345**

17. 12:00 midnight = **2400**

18. 3:30 PM = 3:30 + 12:00 = **1530**

19. 6:20 AM = **0620**

20. 5:45 PM = 5:45 + 12:00 = **1745**

Review Set 16 (page 57)

Formulas

$$°F = 1.8°C + 32° \qquad °C = \frac{°F - 32}{1.8}$$

1. $0°F = \mathbf{-17.8°C}$

$$°C = \frac{°F - 32}{1.8}$$
$$°C = \frac{0 - 32}{1.8}$$
$$°C = \frac{-32}{1.8}$$
$$°C = -17.8$$

$$
\begin{array}{r}
1\,7.77 \\
1.8\overline{)32.0.0} \\
-18 \\
\hline
140 \\
-126 \\
\hline
140 \\
-126 \\
\hline
14
\end{array}
$$

2. $85°C = \mathbf{185°F}$

$$°F = 1.8°C + 32$$
$$°F = 1.8 \times 85 + 32$$
$$°F = 153 + 32$$
$$°F = 185°$$

$$
\begin{array}{r}
1.8 \\
\times 85 \\
\hline
90 \\
144 \\
\hline
153.0
\end{array}
$$

3. $100°C = \mathbf{212°F}$

$°F = 1.8 \times 100 + 32$

$°F = 180 + 32$

$°F = 212°$

$$\begin{array}{r} 1.8 \\ \times 100 \\ \hline 180.0 \end{array}$$

4. $32°C = \mathbf{89.6°F}$

$°F = 1.8 \times 32 + 32$

$°F = 57.6 + 32$

$°F = 89.6°$

$$\begin{array}{r} 32 \\ \times 1.8 \\ \hline 256 \\ 32 \\ \hline 57.6 \end{array}$$

5. $72°F = \mathbf{22.2°C}$

$°C = \frac{72 - 32}{1.8}$

$°C = \frac{40}{1.8}$

$°C = 22.2°$

$$\begin{array}{r} 22.22 \\ 1.8\overline{)\,40.000} \\ -36 \\ \hline 40 \\ -36 \\ \hline 40 \\ -36 \\ \hline 40 \\ -36 \\ \hline 4 \end{array}$$

6. $99°F = \mathbf{37.2°C}$

$°C = \frac{99 - 32}{1.8}$

$°C = \frac{67}{1.8}$

$°C = 37.2°$

$$\begin{array}{r} 37.22 \\ 1.8\overline{)\,67.000} \\ -54 \\ \hline 130 \\ -126 \\ \hline 40 \\ -36 \\ \hline 40 \\ -36 \\ \hline 4 \end{array}$$

7. $103.6°F = \mathbf{39.8°C}$

$°C = \frac{103.6 - 32}{1.8}$

$°C = \frac{71.6}{1.8}$

$°C = 39.8°$

$$\begin{array}{r} 39.77 \\ 1.8\overline{)\,71.600} \\ -54 \\ \hline 176 \\ -162 \\ \hline 140 \\ -126 \\ \hline 140 \\ -126 \\ \hline 14 \end{array}$$

8. $40°C = \mathbf{104°F}$

$°F = 1.8 \times 40 + 32$

$°F = 72 + 32$

$°F = 104°$

$$\begin{array}{r} 1.8 \\ \times 40 \\ \hline 72.0 \end{array}$$

9. $80°C = \mathbf{176°F}$

$°F = 1.8 \times 80 + 32$

$°F = 144 + 32$

$°F = 176°$

$$\begin{array}{r} 1.8 \\ \times 80 \\ \hline 144.0 \end{array}$$

10. 36.4°C = **97.5°F**

$°F = 1.8 \times 36.4 + 32$

$°F = 65.52 + 32$

$°F = 97.5°$

$$\begin{array}{r} 1.8 \\ \times\, 36.4 \\ \hline 72 \\ 108 \\ 54 \\ \hline 65.52 \end{array}$$

11. 100°F = **37.8°C**

$°C = \frac{100 - 32}{1.8}$

$°C = \frac{68}{1.8}$

$°C = 37.8°$

$$\begin{array}{r} 37.77 \\ 1.8\,\overline{)\,68.000} \\ -54 \\ \hline 140 \\ -126 \\ \hline 140 \\ -126 \\ \hline 140 \\ -126 \\ \hline 14 \end{array}$$

12. 19°C = **66.2°F**

$°F = 1.8 \times 19 + 32$

$°F = 34.2 + 32$

$°F = 66.2°$

$$\begin{array}{r} 19 \\ \times 1.8 \\ \hline 152 \\ 19 \\ \hline 34.2 \end{array}$$

13. 4°C = **39.2°F**

$°F = 1.8 \times 4 + 32$

$°F = 7.2 + 32$

$°F = 39.2°$

$$\begin{array}{r} 1.8 \\ \times 4 \\ \hline 7.2 \end{array}$$

14. 94.2°F = **34.6°C**

$°C = \frac{94.2 - 32}{1.8}$

$°C = \frac{62.2}{1.8}$

$°C = 34.6°$

$$\begin{array}{r} 34.55 \\ 1.8\,\overline{)\,62.200} \\ -54 \\ \hline 82 \\ -72 \\ \hline 100 \\ -90 \\ \hline 100 \\ -90 \\ \hline 10 \end{array}$$

15. 102.8°F = **39.3°C**

$°C = \frac{102.8 - 32}{1.8}$

$°C = \frac{70.8}{1.8}$

$°C = 39.3°$

$$\begin{array}{r} 39.33 \\ 1.8\,\overline{)\,70.800} \\ -54 \\ \hline 168 \\ -162 \\ \hline 60 \\ -54 \\ \hline 60 \\ -54 \\ \hline 6 \end{array}$$

Practice Problems—Chapter 3 (page 58)

1. 0.5 g = **500 mg**

$$\frac{1\text{ g}}{1000\text{ mg}} = \frac{0.5\text{ g}}{X\text{ mg}}$$ OR $0.5\text{ g} = 0.5 \times 1000 = 500\text{ mg}$

$$X = 500\text{ mg}$$

2. 0.01 g = **10 mg**

$$\frac{1\text{ g}}{1000\text{ mg}} = \frac{0.01\text{ g}}{X\text{ mg}}$$ OR $0.01\text{ g} = 0.01 \times 1000 = 10\text{ mg}$

$$X = 10\text{ mg}$$

3. 7.5 cc = **7.5 mL**

4. 3 qt = **3 L**

5. 4 mg = **0.004 g**

$$\frac{1\text{ g}}{1000\text{ mg}} = \frac{X\text{ g}}{4\text{ mg}}$$ OR $4\text{ mg} = 4 \div 1000 = 0.004\text{ g}$

$$1000X = 4$$

$$\frac{1000X}{1000} = \frac{4}{1000}$$

$$X = 0.004\text{ g}$$

6. 500 mL = **0.5 L**

$$\frac{1\text{ L}}{1000\text{ mL}} = \frac{X\text{ L}}{500\text{ mL}}$$ OR $500\text{ mL} = 500 \div 1000 = 0.5\text{ L}$

$$1000X = 500$$

$$\frac{1000X}{1000} = \frac{500}{1000}$$

$$X = \frac{1}{2} = 0.5\text{ L}$$

7. 250 mL = **pt ss**

$$\frac{\text{pt i}}{500\text{ mL}} = \frac{\text{pt X}}{250\text{ mL}}$$ OR $250\text{ mL} = 250 \div 500 = \frac{1}{2} = \text{pt ss}$

$$\frac{1}{500} = \frac{X}{250}$$

$$500X = 250$$

$$\frac{500X}{500} = \frac{250}{500}$$

$$X = \frac{1}{2}$$

$$X = \text{pt ss}$$

8. 300 g = **0.3 kg**

$$\frac{1\text{ kg}}{1000\text{ g}} = \frac{X\text{ kg}}{300\text{ g}}$$ OR $300\text{ g} = 300 \div 1000 = 0.3\text{ kg}$

$$1000X = 300$$

$$\frac{1000X}{1000} = \frac{300}{1000}$$

$$X = \frac{3}{10} = 0.3\text{ kg}$$

9. 28 in = **70 cm**

$$\frac{1\text{ in}}{2.5\text{ cm}} = \frac{28\text{ in}}{X\text{ cm}}$$ OR $28\text{ in} = 28 \times 2.5 = 70\text{ cm}$

$$X = 70\text{ cm}$$

$$\begin{array}{r} 28 \\ \times\, 2.5 \\ \hline 140 \\ 56 \\ \hline 70.0 \end{array}$$

10. 68 kg = **149.6 lb**

$$\frac{1\text{ kg}}{2.2\text{ lb}} = \frac{68\text{ kg}}{X\text{ lb}}$$ OR $68\text{ kg} = 68 \times 2.2 = 149.6\text{ lb}$

$$X = 149.6\text{ lb}$$

$$\begin{array}{r} 68 \\ \times\, 2.2 \\ \hline 136 \\ 136 \\ \hline 149.6 \end{array}$$

11. gr iii = **180 mg** $\dfrac{\text{gr i}}{60 \text{ mg}} = \dfrac{\text{gr iii}}{X \text{ mg}}$ OR   gr iii = 3×60 = 180 mg

$\dfrac{1}{60} = \dfrac{3}{X}$

X = 180 mg

12. ℨ iiiss = **105 mL** $\dfrac{ℨ \text{ i}}{30 \text{ mL}} = \dfrac{ℨ \text{ iiiss}}{X \text{ mL}}$ OR   ℨ iiiss = $3\frac{1}{2} \times 30 = \dfrac{7}{\cancel{2}} \times \overset{15}{\cancel{30}}$ = 105 mL

$\dfrac{1}{30} = \dfrac{3.5}{X}$

X = 105 mL

13. gr $\frac{1}{200}$ = **0.3 mg** $\dfrac{\text{gr i}}{60 \text{ mg}} = \dfrac{\text{gr}\frac{1}{200}}{X \text{ mg}}$ OR   gr $\frac{1}{200} = \dfrac{1}{\cancel{200}} \times \cancel{60} = \dfrac{6}{20} = \dfrac{3}{10}$ = 0.3 mg

$X = \dfrac{1}{\cancel{200}} \times \dfrac{\cancel{60}}{1}$

$X = \dfrac{6}{20} = \dfrac{3}{10}$ = 0.3 mg

14. gr $\frac{1}{4}$ = **15 mg** $\dfrac{\text{gr i}}{60 \text{ mg}} = \dfrac{\text{gr}\frac{1}{4}}{X \text{ mg}}$ OR   gr $\frac{1}{4} = \dfrac{1}{\cancel{4}} \times \overset{15}{\cancel{60}}$ = 15 mg

$X = \dfrac{1}{\cancel{4}} \times \overset{15}{\cancel{60}}$

X = 15 mg

15. gr $\frac{1}{10}$ = **6 mg** $\dfrac{\text{gr i}}{60 \text{ mg}} = \dfrac{\text{gr}\frac{1}{10}}{X \text{mg}}$ OR   gr $\frac{1}{10} = \dfrac{1}{\cancel{10}} \times \dfrac{\overset{6}{\cancel{60}}}{1}$ = 6 mg

$X = \dfrac{1}{10} \times 60 = 6$

X = 6 mg

16. gr iss = **90 mg** $\dfrac{\text{gr i}}{60 \text{ mg}} = \dfrac{\text{gr iss}}{X \text{ mg}}$ OR   gr iss = $1\frac{1}{2} \times 60 = \dfrac{3}{\cancel{2}} \times \overset{30}{\cancel{60}}$ = 90 mg

$\dfrac{1}{60} = \dfrac{1.5}{X}$

X = 90 mg

17. $70\frac{1}{2}$ lb = **32.0 kg** $\dfrac{1 \text{ kg}}{2.2 \text{ lb}} = \dfrac{X \text{ kg}}{70\frac{1}{2} \text{ lb}}$ OR $70\frac{1}{2}$ lb = $70.5 \div 2.2$ = 32.0 kg

$2.2X = 70.5$

$\dfrac{2.2X}{2.2} = \dfrac{70.5}{2.2}$

X = 32.0 kg

```
        32.04
2.2)70.500
   -66
   ‾‾‾
     45
    -44
    ‾‾‾
     100
     -88
     ‾‾‾
      12
```

18. 3634 g = **7.9 lb or 8 lb** $\dfrac{1 \text{ kg}}{1000 \text{ g}} = \dfrac{X \text{ kg}}{3634 \text{ g}}$ OR   3634 g = $3634 \div 1000$ = 3.634 or 3.6 kg

$1000X = 3634$

3.6 kg = 3.6×2.2 = 7.92 = 7.9 lb

$\dfrac{1000X}{1000} = \dfrac{3634}{1000}$

X = 3.634

X = 3.6 kg

$\dfrac{1 \text{ kg}}{2.2 \text{ lb}} = \dfrac{3.6 \text{ kg}}{X \text{ lb}}$

X = 7.9 lb

```
   3.6
 ×2.2
 ‾‾‾‾
   72
  72
 ‾‾‾‾
 7.92
```

19. 8 mL = **0.008 L**

$$\frac{1\ L}{1000\ mL} = \frac{X\ L}{8\ mL}$$

$$1000X = 8$$

$$\frac{1000X}{1000} = \frac{8}{1000}$$

$$X = 0.008\ L$$

OR 8 mL = 8 ÷ 1000 = 0.008 L

20. gr xxx = **2 g**

$$\frac{1\ g}{gr\ 15} = \frac{X\ g}{gr\ xxx}$$

$$\frac{1}{15} = \frac{X}{30}$$

$$15X = 30$$

$$\frac{15X}{15} = \frac{30}{15}$$

$$X = 2\ g$$

OR gr xxx = 30 ÷ 15 = 2 g

21. 237.5 cm = **95 in**

$$\frac{1\ in}{2.5\ cm} = \frac{X\ in}{237.5\ cm}$$

$$2.5X = 237.5$$

$$\frac{2.5X}{2.5} = \frac{237.5}{2.5}$$

$$X = 95\ in$$

OR 237.5 cm = 237.5 ÷ 2.5 =

$$\begin{array}{r} 9\ 5 \\ 2.5\overline{)237.5} \\ -225 \\ \hline 125 \\ -125 \\ \hline 0 \end{array}$$

22. 0.5 g = **gr viiss**

$$\frac{1\ g}{gr\ 15} = \frac{0.5\ g}{gr\ X}$$

$$\frac{1}{15} = \frac{0.5}{X}$$

$$X = 7.5$$

$$X = gr\ viiss$$

OR $0.5\ g = \frac{1}{2} \times 15 = \frac{15}{2} = 7\frac{1}{2} = gr\ viiss$

23. 0.6 mg = **gr $\frac{1}{100}$**

$$\frac{gr\ i}{60\ mg} = \frac{gr\ X}{0.6\ mg}$$

$$\frac{1}{60} = \frac{X}{0.6}$$

$$60X = 0.6$$

$$\frac{60X}{60} = \frac{0.6}{60}$$

$$X = \frac{\overset{1}{\cancel{6}}}{10} \times \frac{1}{\underset{10}{\cancel{60}}}$$

$$X = \frac{1}{100}$$

$$X = gr\frac{1}{100}$$

OR $0.6\ mg = \frac{6}{10} \div 60 = \frac{\overset{1}{\cancel{6}}}{10} \times \frac{1}{\underset{10}{\cancel{60}}} = \frac{1}{100} = gr\ \frac{1}{100}$

24. gr x = **0.67 g**

$$\frac{1\ g}{gr\ 15} = \frac{X\ g}{gr\ X}$$

$$\frac{1}{15} = \frac{X}{10}$$

$$15X = 10$$

$$\frac{15X}{15} = \frac{10}{15}$$

$$X = \frac{2}{3}$$

$$X = 0.67\ g$$

OR gr X = 10 ÷ 15 = $\frac{2}{3}$ = 0.67 g

$$\begin{array}{r} 0.666\ldots \\ 3\overline{)2.00} \\ -18 \\ \hline 20 \\ -18 \\ \hline 20 \end{array}$$

25. 150 lb = **68.2 kg** $\dfrac{1\text{ kg}}{2.2\text{ lb}} = \dfrac{X\text{ kg}}{150\text{ lb}}$ OR   150 lb = 150 ÷ 2.2 = 68.2 kg

$2.2X = 150$

$\dfrac{2.2X}{2.2} = \dfrac{150}{2.2}$

$X = 68.2\text{ kg}$

$$\begin{array}{r} 68.18 \\ 2.2\overline{)150.0} \\ -132 \\ \hline 180 \\ -176 \\ \hline 40 \\ -22 \\ \hline 180 \\ -176 \\ \hline 4 \end{array}$$

26. 60 mg = **gr i**

27. gr 15 = **1 g**

28. 2 cups = **500 cc** $\dfrac{1\text{ cup}}{250\text{ cc}} = \dfrac{2\text{ cups}}{X\text{ cc}}$ OR   2 cups = 2 × 250 = 500 cc

$X = 500\text{ cc}$

29. 6 t = **2 T** $\dfrac{1\text{ T}}{3\text{ t}} = \dfrac{X\text{ T}}{6\text{ t}}$ OR   6 t = 6 ÷ 3 = 2 T

$3X = 6$

$\dfrac{3X}{3} = \dfrac{6}{3}$

$X = 2\text{ T}$

30. $\dfrac{℥\text{ i}}{30\text{ mL}} = \dfrac{℥\text{ X}}{90\text{ mL}}$ OR   90 mL = 90 ÷ 30 = 3 = ℥ iii

$\dfrac{1}{30} = \dfrac{X}{90}$

$30X = 90$

$\dfrac{30X}{30} = \dfrac{90}{30}$

$X = 3$

X = ℥ iii

31. 1 ft = **12 in** $\dfrac{1\text{ in}}{2.5\text{ cm}} = \dfrac{12\text{ in}}{X\text{ cm}}$ OR   12 in = 12 × 2.5 = 30 cm

$X = \textbf{30 cm}$

$$\begin{array}{r} 2.5 \\ \times 12 \\ \hline 50 \\ 25 \\ \hline 30.0 \end{array}$$

32. $\dfrac{1\text{ T}}{15\text{ cc}} = \dfrac{2\text{ T}}{X\text{ cc}}$ OR   2 T = 2 × 15 = 30 cc

$X = \textbf{30 cc}$

33. 2.2 lb. = **1 kg**

34. 5 cc = **1 t**

35. 1000 mL = **1 L**

36. 1.5 g = **1500 mg** $\dfrac{1\text{ g}}{1000\text{ mg}} = \dfrac{1.5\text{ g}}{X\text{ mg}}$ OR   1.5 g = 1.5 × 1000 = 1500 mg

$X = 1500\text{ mg}$

$1.5 \times 1000 = 1.500 \times 1000 = 1500$

37. ℥ iss = **45 cc**

$$\frac{℥\ i}{30\ cc} = \frac{℥\ iss}{X\ cc}$$

$$\frac{1}{30} = \frac{1.5}{X}$$

$$X = 45\ cc$$

OR

℥ iss = 1.5 × 30 = 45 cc

$$\begin{array}{r} 1.5 \\ \times\,30 \\ \hline 45.0 \end{array}$$

38. 1500 mL = **qt iss**

$$\frac{qt\ i}{1000\ mL} = \frac{qt\ X}{1500\ mL}$$

$$\frac{1}{1000} = \frac{X}{1500}$$

$$1000X = 1500$$

$$\frac{1000X}{1000} = \frac{1500}{1000}$$

$$X = 1.5$$

$$X = qt\ iss$$

OR

1500 mL = 1500 ÷ 1000 = 1.5 = qt iss

39. 10 mg = **gr $\frac{1}{6}$**

$$\frac{gr\ i}{60\ mg} = \frac{gr\ X}{10\ mg}$$

$$\frac{1}{60} = \frac{X}{10}$$

$$60X = 10$$

$$\frac{60X}{60} = \frac{10}{60}$$

$$X = \frac{1}{6}$$

$$X = gr\ \frac{1}{6}$$

OR

10 mg = 10 ÷ 60 = $\frac{1}{6}$ = gr $\frac{1}{6}$

40. 25 mg = **0.025 g**

$$\frac{1\ g}{1000\ mg} = \frac{X\ g}{25\ mg}$$

$$1000X = 25$$

$$\frac{1000X}{1000} = \frac{25}{1000}$$

$$X = 0.025\ g$$

OR

25 mg = 25 ÷ 1000 = 0.025 g

41. 4.3 kg = **4300 g**

$$\frac{1\ kg}{1000\ g} = \frac{4.3\ kg}{X\ g}$$

$$X = 4300\ g$$

OR

4.3 kg = 4.3 × 1000 = 4300 g

4.3 × 1000 = 4.300 × 1000 = 4300

42. 60 mg = **0.06 g**

$$\frac{1\ g}{1000\ mg} = \frac{X\ g}{60\ mg}$$

$$1000X = 60$$

$$\frac{1000X}{1000} = \frac{60}{1000}$$

$$X = 0.06\ g$$

OR

60 mg = 60 ÷ 1000 = 0.06 g

60 ÷ 1000 = 0060. ÷ 1000 = 0.06

43. 0.015 g = **15 mg**

$$\frac{1\ g}{1000\ mg} = \frac{0.015\ g}{X\ mg}$$

$$X = 15\ mg$$

OR

0.015 g = 0.015 × 1000 = 15 mg

0.015 × 1000 = 15

44. 45 cc = **45 mL**

45. gr 12 = **0.8 g**

$$\frac{1\,g}{gr\,15} = \frac{X\,g}{gr\,12}$$

$$\frac{1}{15} = \frac{X}{12}$$

$$15X = 12$$

$$\frac{15X}{15} = \frac{12}{15}$$

$$X = \frac{4}{5} \text{ or } 0.8$$

OR

gr 12 = 12 ÷ 15 = $\frac{4}{5}$ = 0.8

$$5)\overline{4.0} \quad \begin{array}{r} 0.8 \\ \end{array}$$

$$\begin{array}{r} -40 \\ \hline 0 \end{array}$$

46. 3.6 g = **3,600 mg**

$$\frac{1\,g}{1000\,mg} = \frac{3.6\,g}{X\,mg}$$

$$X = 3600\,mg$$

OR

3.6 g = 3.6 × 1000 = 3600 g

$$3.6 \times 1000 = 3.600 \times 1000 = 3600$$

47. 3.6 mg = **0.0036 g**

$$\frac{1\,g}{1000\,mg} = \frac{X\,g}{3.6\,mg}$$

$$1000X = 3.6$$

$$\frac{1000X}{1000} = \frac{3.6}{1000}$$

$$X = 0.0036\,g$$

OR

3.6 mg = 3.6 ÷ 1000 = 0.0036 g

$$3.6 \div 1000 = 0003.6 \div 1000 = 0.0036$$

48. 10 mL = **0.01 L**

$$\frac{1\,L}{1000\,mL} = \frac{X\,L}{10\,mL}$$

$$1000X = 10$$

$$\frac{1000X}{1000} = \frac{10}{1000}$$

$$X = 0.01\,L$$

OR

10 mL = 10 ÷ 1000 = 0.01 L

$$10 \div 1000 = 0010. \div 1000 = 0.01$$

49. 2 t = **10 mL**

$$\frac{1\,t}{5\,mL} = \frac{2\,t}{X\,mL}$$

$$X = 10\,mL$$

OR

2 t = 2 × 5 = 10 mL

50. 170 mg = **0.17 g**

$$\frac{1\,g}{1000\,mg} = \frac{X\,g}{170\,mg}$$

$$1000X = 170$$

$$\frac{1000X}{1000} = \frac{170}{1000}$$

$$X = 0.17\,g$$

OR

170 mg = 170 ÷ 1000 = 0.17 g

$$170. \div 1000 = 0.17$$

51. 1730 = 1730 − 1200 = **5:30 PM**

52. 8:30 PM = 8:30 + 12:00 = **2030**

53. 0915 = **9:15 AM**

54. 98°F = **36.7°C**

$$°C = \frac{98 - 32}{1.8}$$

$$°C = \frac{66}{1.8}$$

$$°C = 36.66\ldots$$

$$°C = 36.7°$$

$$1.8)\overline{660.00} \quad \begin{array}{r} 36.66 \\ \end{array}$$

$$\begin{array}{r} -54 \\ \hline 120 \\ -108 \\ \hline 120 \\ -108 \\ \hline 120 \\ -108 \end{array}$$

55. 110°C = **230°F**

$$°F = 1.8 \times 110 + 32$$
$$°F = 198 + 32$$
$$°F = 230°$$

$$\begin{array}{r} 110 \\ \times 1.8 \\ \hline 880 \\ 110 \\ \hline 198.0 \end{array}$$

56. 30°C = **86°F**

$$°F = 1.8 \times 30 + 32$$
$$°F = 54 + 32$$
$$°F = 86°$$

$$\begin{array}{r} 30 \\ \times 1.8 \\ \hline 240 \\ 30 \\ \hline 54.0 \end{array}$$

57. 2°F = **−16.7°C**

$$°C = \frac{2 - 32}{1.8}$$
$$°C = -\frac{30}{1.8}$$
$$°C = 16.66°\ldots$$

$$\begin{array}{r} 16.66 \\ 1.8\overline{)30.000} \\ -18 \\ \hline 120 \\ -108 \\ \hline 120 \\ -108 \\ \hline 120 \\ -108 \\ \hline 120 \end{array}$$

58. 2001 = 2001 − 1200 = **8:01 PM**

59. 7:30 PM = 7:30 + 12:00 = **1930**

60. 6:45 AM = **0645**

61. 12 midnight = 12:00 + 12:00 = **2400**

62.

$$\frac{3\,i}{6\,t} = \frac{3\,iv}{X\,t}$$

$$\frac{1}{6} = \frac{4}{X}$$

X = 24 t in bottle

$$\frac{1\ dose}{2\frac{1}{2}\,t} = \frac{X\ doses}{24\,t}$$

$$2\frac{1}{2}X = 24$$

$$\frac{2\frac{1}{2}X}{2\frac{1}{2}} = \frac{24}{2\frac{1}{2}}$$

$$X = 24 \div 2\frac{1}{2}$$

$$X = 24 \div \frac{5}{2}$$

$$X = 24 \times \frac{2}{5}$$

$$X = \frac{48}{5}$$

$$X = 9\frac{3}{5}\ \text{or } \textbf{9 complete doses}$$

63. 1 T = 15 mL

$$\frac{1\ T}{15\ mL} = \frac{X\ T}{120\ mL}$$

$$15X = 120$$

$$\frac{15X}{15} = \frac{120}{15}$$

$$X = 8\ T = \textbf{8 doses}$$

$$15\overline{)120} \quad \begin{array}{r} 8 \\ -120 \\ \hline 0 \end{array}$$

64. 4 ounces

     8 ounces

     6 ounces

     10 ounces

    ----

     28 ounces

$$\frac{\mathfrak{Z}\ i}{30\ mL} = \frac{\mathfrak{Z}\ 28}{X\ mL}$$

$$X = \textbf{840 mL}$$

$$\begin{array}{r} 30 \\ \times 28 \\ \hline 240 \\ 60 \\ \hline 840 \end{array}$$

65. $\dfrac{gr\ i}{60\ mg} = \dfrac{gr\frac{1}{6}}{X\ mg}$

$$X = \frac{1}{\cancel{6}} \times \cancel{60}^{\,10} = 10\ mg = 1\ \text{full ampule}$$

You will administer **100%** of the ampule

Review Set 17 (page 69)

1. **tuberculin syringe**

2. a. **yes**

   b. **Round 1.25 mL to 1.3 mL and measure on the cc scale as 1.3 cc.**

3. **No**

4. $\dfrac{1 \text{ cc}}{100 \text{ U}} = \dfrac{X \text{ cc}}{50 \text{ U}}$

   $100X = 50$

   $\dfrac{100X}{100} = \dfrac{50}{100}$

   $X = \textbf{0.5 cc}$

5. a. **False**

   b. **The size of the drop varies according to the diameter of the dropper.**

6. **No**

7. **Measure the oral liquid in a needleless 3 cc syringe.**

8. **5 mL**

9. **Discard the excess prior to injecting the patient.**

10. **To prevent needlestick injury.**

11. **Administer 0.75 cc**

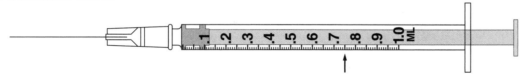

12. **Administer 1.33 cc**

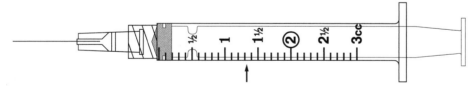

13. **Administer 2.2 cc**

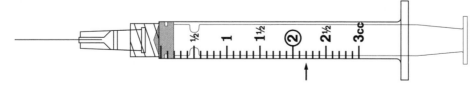

14. **Administer 1.3 cc**

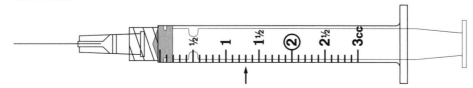

15. **Administer 0.33 cc**

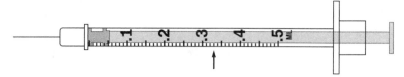

16. **Administer 66 U of U-100 insulin**

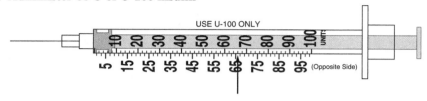

17. **Administer 27 U of U-100 insulin**

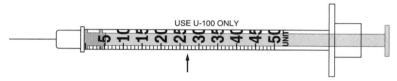

18. **Administer 75 U of U-100 insulin**

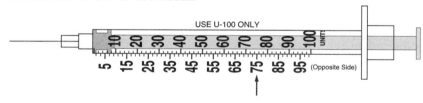

19. **Administer 4.4 cc**

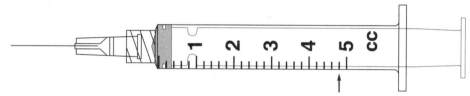

20. **Administer 16 cc**

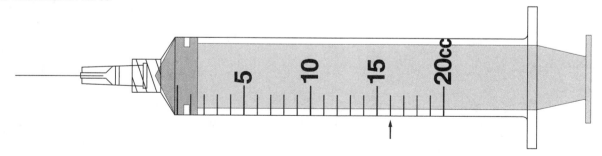

Practice Problems—Chapter 4 (page 72)

1. 100 U = **1 cc**

2. **hundredths**

3. **No, a tuberculin syringe only measures a total of 1 mL. You would need two tuberculin syringes to measure 1.25 cc.**

4. **Round to 1.3 mL and measure 1.3 mL.**

5. **30 mL or 1 ounce capacity**

6. **1 mL tuberculin**

7. $\dfrac{1\,cc}{100\,U} = \dfrac{X\,cc}{75\,U}$

   $100X = 75$

   $\dfrac{100X}{100} = \dfrac{75}{100}$

      $X = \mathbf{0.75\ cc}$

8. **False**

9. **False**

10. **True**

11. **Administer 0.45 mL**

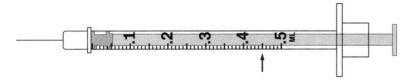

12. **Administer 80 U of U-100 syringe**

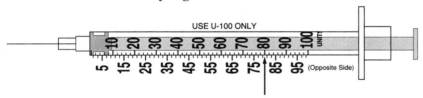

13. **Administer 2 t**

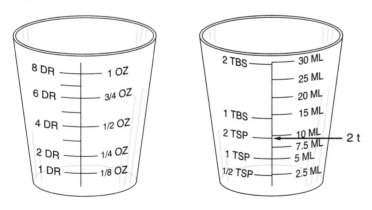

14. **Administer 2.4 mL**

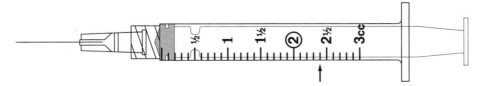

15. **Administer 1.1 mL**

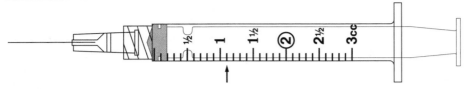

16. **Administer 6.2 mL**

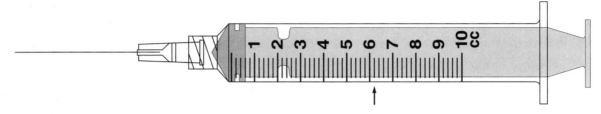

Review Set 18 (page 79)

1. **6 AM, 12 noon, 6 PM, 12 midnight**

2. **9 AM**

3. **7:30 AM, 11:30 AM, 4:30 PM, 9 PM**

4. **9 AM, 5 PM**

5. **every 4 hours, as needed**

6. **9/7/xx at 0900 (9 AM)**

7. **Sublingual (under the tongue)**

8. **once a day**

9. $$\frac{1\,mg}{1000\,mcg} = \frac{0.125\,mg}{X}$$
   $$X = 0.125 \times 1000$$
   $$X = 125\,mcg$$

10. **nitroglycerin**
    Darvocet-N 100
    meperidine (Demerol)
    promethazine (Phenergan)

11. **subcutaneous injection**

12. **once (at 9 AM)**

13. **Keflex**

14. **before breakfast (at 7:30 AM)**

15. **milliequivalent**

16. **Keflex and Slow K**

17. **Tylenol**

18. **twice (at 9 AM and 9 PM)**

19. **0900 and 2100**

20. **2400, 0600, 1200, and 1800**

21. **In the "One Time Medication Dosage" section, lower left corner.**

Review Set 19 (page 82)

1. **Give 250 mg of naproxen orally two times a day.**

2. **Give 30 units of Humulin N U-100 insulin subcutaneously every day 30 minutes before breakfast.**

3. **Give 500 mg or Ceclor orally immediately and then give 250 mg every eight hours.**

4. **Give 25 micrograms of Synthroid orally once a day.**

5. **Give 10 milligrams of Ativan intramuscularly every 4 hours as necessary for agitation.**

6. **Give 20 milligrams of furosemide intravenously (slowly) immediately.**

7. **Give 10 cubic centimeters of Gelusil orally at bed time.**

8. **Give 2 drops of 1% atropine sulfate ophthalmic in the right eye every 15 minutes for four applications.**

9. **Give $\frac{1}{4}$ grain of morphine sulfate intramuscularly every three to four hours as needed for pain.**

10. **Give 0.25 milligrams of Lanoxin orally once a day.**

11. **Give 250 milligrams of tetracycline orally four times a day.**

12. **Give $\frac{1}{400}$ grain of nitroglycerin sublingually immediately.**

13. **Give 2 drops Cortisporin Otic in both ears three times a day and at bedtime.**

14. **1, 6, 8, 9, 11, 12.**

15. **Contact the physician for clarification.**

16. **No; q.i.d. is given only 4 times during 24 hours, whereas q.4h is given 6 times in 24 hours.**

17. **Determined by the policy at the facility, and the drug order.**

18. **Patient, drug, dosage, route, frequency, date and time, signature of doctor/writer.**

19. **Parts 1–5**

20. **The right patient must receive the right drug in the right amount by the right route at the right time.**

Practice Problems—Chapter 5 (page 85)

1. **ounce**

2. **per rectum**

3. **before meals**

4. **after**

5. **three times a day**

6. **every four hours**

7. **when necessary**

8. **by mouth, orally**

9. **once a day, every day**

10. **right eye**

11. **immediately**

12. **freely (as desired)**

13. **hour of sleep (at bedtime)**

14. **intramuscular**

15. **without**

16. **ss**

17. **gtt**

18. **mL**

19. **gr**

20. **g**

21. **c̄**

22. **q.i.d.**

23. **O.U.**

24. **SC**

25. **t**

26. **b.i.d.**

27. **q.3h**

28. **p.c.**

29. **ā**

30. **kg**

31. **Give 60 milligrams of Toradol intramuscularly immediately and then every six hours.**

32. **Give 300,000 units of procaine penicillin G intramuscularly four times a day.**

33. **Give 5 milliliters of Mylanta orally one hour before meals, 1 hour after meals, at bedtime, and every two hours when necessary at night.**

34. **Give 25 milligrams of Librium orally every six hours when necessary for agitation.**

35. **Give 5,000 units of heparin subcutaneously immediately.**

36. **Give 50 milligrams of Demerol intramuscularly every 3–4 hours when necessary for pain.**

37. **Give 0.25 milligrams of digoxin by mouth every day.**

38. **Give 2 drops of 10% Neosynephrine ophthalmic to the left eye every thirty minutes for 2 applications.**

39. **Give 40 milligrams of Lasix intramuscularly immediately.**

40. **Give 4 milligrams of Decadron intravenously twice a day.**

41. **12 midnight, 8 AM, 4 PM**

42. **20 units**

43. **SC (subcutaneous)**

44. **Give 500 mg Cipro orally every 12 hours.**

45. **8:00 AM, 12:00 noon, 6:00 PM**

46. **Digoxin 0.125 mg po. q.d.**

47. **with, c̄**

48. **Give 150 mg of ranitidine orally twice a day with breakfast and supper**

49. **Vancomycin**

50. **12 hours**

Review Set 20 (page 94)

1. **B**

2. **D**

3. **C**

4. **A**

5. **E**

6. **F**

7. **G**

8. **1 capsule**

9. **For IM or IV injection use.**

Practice Problems—Chapter 6 (page 97)

1. **1 tablet = 8 mEq**

2. **Summit Pharmaceuticals—Division of CIBA-Geigy Corporation**

3. **ampicillin sodium/sulbactam sodium**

4. **Reconstitute with up to 100 mL of an appropriate diluent cited in the package insert.**

5. **10 mL**

6. **25 mg/mL**

7. **Keflin**

8. **cephalothin sodium**

9. **fluid intramuscular solution**

10. **10 mL**

11. **Roche Laboratories**

12. **capsule**

13. **4/00 April 2000**

14. **1 tablet = 80 mg**

15. **J**

16. **H**

17. **H**

18. **po (oral)**

19. **0666060**

20. **80 mg tablet**

Review Set 21 (page 109)

1. $0.1 \text{ g} = 0.1 \times 1000 = 100 \text{ mg}$

    $$\frac{100 \text{ mg}}{1 \text{ tab}} = \frac{100 \text{ mg}}{\text{X tab}}$$

    $$100\text{X} = 100$$

    $$\frac{100\text{X}}{100} = \frac{100}{100}$$

    $$\text{X} = \textbf{1 tablet}$$

2. $0.5 \text{ g} = 0.5 \times 1000 = 500 \text{ mg}$

    $$\frac{500 \text{ mg}}{1 \text{ tab}} = \frac{500 \text{ mg}}{\text{X tab}}$$

    $$500\text{X} = 500$$

    $$\frac{500\text{X}}{500} = \frac{500}{500}$$

    $$\text{X} = \textbf{1 tablet}$$

3. $$\frac{10 \text{ mg}}{1 \text{ tab}} = \frac{15 \text{ mg}}{\text{X tab}}$$

    $$10\text{X} = 15$$

    $$\frac{10\text{X}}{10} = \frac{15}{10}$$

    $$\text{X} = 1.5 = \textbf{1}\frac{\textbf{1}}{\textbf{2}} \textbf{ tablets}$$

4. $$\frac{25 \text{ mg}}{1 \text{ tab}} = \frac{12.5 \text{ mg}}{\text{X tab}}$$

    $$25\text{X} = 12.5$$

    $$\frac{25\text{X}}{25} = \frac{12.5}{25}$$

    $$\text{X} = \frac{\textbf{1}}{\textbf{2}} \textbf{ tablet}$$

    $$\begin{array}{r} 0.5 \\ 25\overline{)12.5} \\ -125 \\ \hline 0 \end{array}$$

5. $$\frac{0.25 \text{ mg}}{1 \text{ tab}} = \frac{0.125 \text{ mg}}{\text{X tab}}$$

    $$0.25\text{X} = 0.125$$

    $$\frac{0.25\text{X}}{0.25} = \frac{0.125}{0.25}$$

    $$\text{X} = \frac{\textbf{1}}{\textbf{2}} \textbf{ tablet}$$

    $$\begin{array}{r} 0.5 \\ 0.25\overline{)0.125} \\ -125 \\ \hline 0 \end{array}$$

6. $$\frac{300 \text{ mg}}{1 \text{ tab}} = \frac{600 \text{ mg}}{\text{X tab}}$$

    $$300\text{X} = 600$$

    $$\frac{300\text{X}}{300} = \frac{600}{300}$$

    $$\text{X} = \textbf{2 tablets}$$

7. $$\frac{8 \text{ mEq}}{1 \text{ tab}} = \frac{16 \text{ mEq}}{\text{X tab}}$$

    $$8\text{X} = 16$$

    $$\frac{8\text{X}}{8} = \frac{16}{8}$$

    $$\text{X} = \textbf{2 tablets}$$

8. $$\frac{25 \text{ mg}}{1 \text{ tab}} = \frac{50 \text{ mg}}{\text{X tab}}$$

    $$25\text{X} = 50$$

    $$\frac{25\text{X}}{25} = \frac{50}{25}$$

    $$\text{X} = \textbf{2 tablets}$$

9. $$\frac{5 \text{ mg}}{1 \text{ tab}} = \frac{7.5 \text{ mg}}{\text{X tab}}$$

    $$5\text{X} = 7.5$$

    $$\frac{5\text{X}}{5} = \frac{7.5}{5}$$

    $$\text{X} = 1\frac{\textbf{1}}{\textbf{2}} \textbf{ tablets}$$

    $$\begin{array}{r} 1.5 \\ 5\overline{)7.5} \\ -5 \\ \hline 25 \\ \hline 0 \end{array}$$

10. $4 \text{ g} = 4 \times 1000 = 4000 \text{ mg}$

    $$\frac{500 \text{ mg}}{1 \text{ tab}} = \frac{4000 \text{ mg}}{\text{X tab}}$$

    $$500\text{X} = 4000$$

    $$\frac{500\text{X}}{500} = \frac{4000}{500}$$

    $$\text{X} = \textbf{8 tablets}$$

11. $$\frac{1 \text{ kg}}{2.2 \text{ lb}} = \frac{\text{X kg}}{145 \text{ lb}}$$

    $$2.2\text{X} = 145$$

    $$\frac{2.2\text{X}}{2.2} = \frac{145}{2.2}$$

    $$\text{X} = 65.9 \text{ kg}$$

    per day,

    $$\frac{0.06 \text{ g}}{1 \text{ kg}} = \frac{\text{X g}}{65.9 \text{ kg}}$$

    $$\text{X} = 4 \text{ g (daily dosage)}$$

    $$\begin{array}{r} 65.90 \\ 2.2\overline{)145.000} \\ -132 \\ \hline 130 \\ -110 \\ \hline 200 \\ -198 \\ \hline 20 \end{array}$$

    $$\begin{array}{r} 65.9 \\ \times 0.06 \\ \hline 3.954 \text{ or } 4.0 \end{array}$$

    Individual q.i.d. dose $= \frac{4 \text{ g}}{4} = 1$ g per dose

    $$\frac{0.5 \text{ g}}{1 \text{ tab}} = \frac{1 \text{ g}}{\text{X tab}}$$

    $$0.5\text{X} = 1$$

    $$\frac{0.5\text{X}}{0.5} = \frac{1}{0.5}$$

    $$\text{X} = \textbf{2 tablets}$$

    $$\begin{array}{r} 2 \\ 0.5\overline{)1.0} \\ -10 \\ \hline 0 \end{array}$$

12. $$\frac{300 \text{ mg}}{1 \text{ tab}} = \frac{150 \text{ mg}}{\text{X tab}}$$

    $$300\text{X} = 150$$

    $$\frac{300\text{X}}{300} = \frac{150}{300}$$

    $$\text{X} = \frac{\textbf{1}}{\textbf{2}} \textbf{ tablet}$$

13.　　1 g = 1000 mg

$$\frac{500 \text{ mg}}{1 \text{ cap}} = \frac{1000 \text{ mg}}{\text{X cap}}$$

$$500\text{X} = 1000$$

$$\frac{500\text{X}}{500} = \frac{1000}{500}$$

X = **2 capsules**

14.　$\frac{1 \text{ mg}}{1000 \text{ mcg}} = \frac{0.05 \text{ mg}}{\text{X mcg}}$

$$\text{X} = 0.05 \times 1000$$

$$\text{X} = 50 \text{ mcg ordered}$$

$$\frac{50 \text{ mcg}}{1 \text{ tab}} = \frac{50 \text{ mcg}}{\text{X tab}}$$

$$50\text{X} = 50$$

$$\frac{50\text{X}}{50} = \frac{50}{50}$$

X = **1 tablet**

15.　$\frac{3.75 \text{ mg}}{1 \text{ cap}} = \frac{7.5 \text{ mg}}{\text{X cap}}$

$$3.75\text{X} = 7.5$$

$$\frac{3.75\text{X}}{3.75} = \frac{7.5}{3.75}$$

X = **2 capsules**

$$3.75\overline{)7.50} \quad \begin{array}{r} 2 \\ \hline -750 \\ \hline 0 \end{array}$$

16.　$\frac{10 \text{ mg}}{\text{tab}} = \frac{15 \text{ mg}}{\text{X tab}}$

$$10\text{X} = 15$$

$$\frac{10\text{X}}{10} = \frac{15}{10} = \frac{3}{2} = 1\frac{1}{2}$$

X = **$1\frac{1}{2}$ tablets**

17.　$\frac{\text{gr i}}{60 \text{ mg}} = \frac{\text{gr}\frac{1}{6}}{\text{X mg}}$

$$\text{X} = \frac{1}{\cancel{6}} \times \cancel{60}^{10}$$

$$\text{X} = 10 \text{ mg}$$

Select 10 mg tablets and give 1 tablet.

18.　$\frac{\text{gr i}}{60 \text{ mg}} = \frac{\text{gr ss}}{\text{X mg}}$

$$\frac{1}{60} = \frac{\frac{1}{2}}{\text{X}}$$

$$\text{X} = \frac{1}{2} \times 60 = 30 \text{ mg}$$

1 h a.c et h.s. = 4 doses in 24 hours

Select 20 mg tablets and give $1\frac{1}{2}$ tablets or give 1-10 mg tablet and 1-20 mg tablet for each dose.

The patient will receive **4 doses** in 24 hours.

19.　$\frac{\text{gr i}}{60 \text{ mg}} = \frac{\text{gr}\frac{1}{4}}{\text{X mg}}$

$$\text{X} = \frac{1}{\cancel{4}} \times \cancel{60}^{15}$$

$$\text{X} = 15 \text{ mg}$$

Select 15 mg tablets and give 1 tablet.

20.　gr i = 60 mg

Select Tylenol with codeine 60 mg tablets and give 1 tablet.

Patient should receive the medication **every 4 hours (q4h) or when necessary for pain.**

21.　**Select label B.**

$$\frac{40 \text{ mg}}{1 \text{ cap}} = \frac{80 \text{ mg}}{\text{X cap}}$$

$$40\text{X} = 80$$

$$\frac{40\text{X}}{40} = \frac{80}{40}$$

X = **2 capsules**

22.　**Select label K.**

$$\frac{1 \text{ g}}{1000 \text{ mg}} = \frac{0.2 \text{ g}}{\text{X mg}}$$

$$\text{X} = 0.2 \times 1000 = 200 \text{ mg}$$

$$\frac{200 \text{ mg}}{1 \text{ tab}} = \frac{200 \text{ mg}}{\text{X tab}}$$

$$200\text{X} = 200$$

$$\frac{200\text{X}}{200} = \frac{200}{200}$$

X = **1 tablet**

23.　**Select label F.**

$$\frac{50 \text{ mg}}{1 \text{ tab}} = \frac{50 \text{ mg}}{\text{X tab}}$$

$$50\text{X} = 50$$

$$\frac{50\text{X}}{50} = \frac{50}{50}$$

X = **1 tablet**

24.　**Select label I.**

$$\frac{8 \text{ mEq}}{1 \text{ tab}} = \frac{16 \text{ mEq}}{\text{X tab}}$$

$$8\text{X} = 16$$

$$\frac{8\text{X}}{8} = \frac{16}{8}$$

X = **2 tablets**

25. Select label C.

$$1 \text{ g} = 1000 \text{ mg}$$

$$\frac{1000 \text{ mg}}{1 \text{ tab}} = \frac{1000 \text{ mg}}{X \text{ tab}}$$

$$1000X = 1000$$

$$\frac{1000X}{1000} = \frac{1000}{1000}$$

$$X = \textbf{1 tablet}$$

26.   Select label E.

$$\frac{1 \text{ g}}{1000 \text{ mg}} = \frac{0.5 \text{ g}}{X \text{ mg}}$$

$$X = 0.5 \times 1000 = 500 \text{ mg}$$

$$\frac{250 \text{ mg}}{1 \text{ cap}} = \frac{500 \text{ mg}}{X \text{ cap}}$$

$$250X = 500$$

$$\frac{250X}{250} = \frac{500}{250}$$

$$X = \textbf{2 capsules}$$

27. Select label D.

$$\frac{1 \text{ g}}{1000 \text{ mg}} = \frac{0.4 \text{ g}}{X \text{ mg}}$$

$$X = 0.4 \times 1000 = 400 \text{ mg}$$

$$\frac{200 \text{ mg}}{1 \text{ cap}} = \frac{400 \text{ mg}}{X \text{ cap}}$$

$$200X = 400$$

$$\frac{200X}{200} = \frac{400}{200}$$

$$X = \textbf{2 capsules}$$

28. Select label H.

$$\frac{0.25 \text{ mg}}{1 \text{ tab}} = \frac{0.5 \text{ mg}}{X \text{ tab}}$$

$$0.25X = 0.5$$

$$\frac{0.25X}{0.25} = \frac{0.5}{0.25}$$

$$X = \textbf{2 tablets}$$

$$0.25 \overline{)0.50} \atop \underline{-50} \atop 0 \quad {}^{2}$$

29. Select label A.

$$\frac{1 \text{ g}}{1000 \text{ mg}} = \frac{0.1 \text{ g}}{X \text{ mg}}$$

$$X = 0.1 \times 1000 = 100 \text{ mg}$$

$$\frac{100 \text{ mg}}{1 \text{ cap}} = \frac{100 \text{ mg}}{X \text{ cap}}$$

$$100X = 100$$

$$\frac{100X}{100} = \frac{100}{100}$$

$$X = \textbf{1 capsule}$$

30. Weight:

$$\frac{1 \text{ kg}}{2.2 \text{ lb}} = \frac{X \text{ kg}}{176 \text{ lb}}$$

$$2.2X = 176$$

$$\frac{2.2X}{2.2} = \frac{176}{2.2}$$

$$X = 80 \text{ kg}$$

$$2.2 \overline{)176.0} \atop \underline{-176} \atop 00 \quad {}^{8\,0}$$

per day,

$$\frac{50 \text{ mg}}{1 \text{ kg}} = \frac{X \text{ mg}}{80 \text{ kg}}$$

$$X = 4000 \text{ mg}$$

per dose,

$$\frac{4000 \text{ mg}}{4 \text{ doses}} = \frac{X \text{ mg}}{\text{dose}}$$

$$4X = 4000$$

$$\frac{4X}{4} = \frac{4000}{4}$$

$$X = 1000 \text{ mg}$$

Select label C.

$$\frac{1000 \text{ mg}}{1 \text{ tab}} = \frac{1000 \text{ mg}}{X \text{ tab}}$$

$$1000X = 1000$$

$$\frac{1000X}{1000} = \frac{1000}{1000}$$

$$X = \textbf{1 tablet for each dose.}$$

Review Set 22 (page 117)

1. $$\frac{50 \text{ mg}}{5 \text{ mL}} = \frac{75 \text{ mg}}{X \text{ mL}}$$

$$50X = 375$$

$$\frac{50X}{50} = \frac{375}{50}$$

$$X = \textbf{7.5 mL}$$

$$50 \overline{)375.0} \atop \underline{-350} \atop 250 \atop \underline{-250} \atop 0 \quad {}^{7.5}$$

2. $$\frac{\text{gr i}}{60 \text{ mg}} = \frac{\text{gr} \frac{1}{6}}{X \text{ mg}}$$

$$X = \frac{1}{\overset{}{6}} \times \overset{10}{\cancel{60}} = 10 \text{ mg}$$

$$\frac{10 \text{ mg}}{5 \text{ mL}} = \frac{10 \text{ mg}}{X \text{ mL}}$$

$$10X = 50$$

$$\frac{10X}{10} = \frac{50}{10}$$

$$X = \textbf{5 mL}$$

3.　　　$1 \text{ g} = 1000 \text{ mg}$

$$\frac{250 \text{ mg}}{5 \text{ mL}} = \frac{1000 \text{ mg}}{X \text{ mL}}$$

$250X = 5000$

$$\frac{250X}{250} = \frac{5000}{250}$$

$X = \textbf{20 mL}$

4.　$\frac{125 \text{ mg}}{5 \text{ mL}} = \frac{100 \text{ mg}}{X \text{ mL}}$

$125X = 500$

$$\frac{125X}{125} = \frac{500}{125}$$

$X = \textbf{4 mL}$

$$125 \overline{)500} \quad \substack{4 \\ -500 \\ \hline 0}$$

5.　$\frac{1 \text{ g}}{1000 \text{ mg}} = \frac{0.5 \text{ g}}{X \text{ mg}}$

$X = 0.5 \times 1000 = 500 \text{ mg}$

$$\frac{500 \text{ mg}}{5 \text{ mL}} = \frac{500 \text{ mg}}{X \text{ mL}}$$

$500X = 2500$

$$\frac{500X}{500} = \frac{2500}{500}$$

$X = 5 \text{ mL}$

$1 \text{ t} = 5 \text{ mL}$ **Give 1 t**

6.　　　$1 \text{ t} = 5 \text{ mL}$

$$\frac{6.25 \text{ mg}}{5 \text{ mL}} = \frac{25 \text{ mg}}{X \text{ mL}}$$

$6.25X = 125$

$$\frac{6.25X}{6.25} = \frac{125}{6.25}$$

$X = \textbf{20 mL}$

$$6.25 \overline{)125.00} \quad \substack{20 \\ -1250 \\ \hline 00}$$

7.　　$5 \text{ mL} = 1 \text{ t}$

$$\frac{62.5 \text{ mg}}{1 \text{ t}} = \frac{125 \text{ mg}}{X \text{ t}}$$

$62.5X = 125$

$$\frac{62.5X}{62.5} = \frac{125}{62.5}$$

$X = \textbf{2 t}$

$$62.5 \overline{)125.0} \quad \substack{2 \\ -1250 \\ \hline 0}$$

8. **Select label B.**

$$\frac{250 \text{ mg}}{5 \text{ mL}} = \frac{125 \text{ mg}}{X \text{ mL}}$$

$250X = 625$

$$\frac{250X}{250} = \frac{625}{250}$$

$X = \textbf{2.5 mL}$

$$250 \overline{)625.0} \quad \substack{2.5 \\ -500 \\ \hline 1250 \\ -1250 \\ \hline 0}$$

9. **Select label C.**

$$\frac{125 \text{ mg}}{5 \text{ mL}} = \frac{50 \text{ mg}}{X \text{ mL}}$$

$125X = 250$

$$\frac{125X}{125} = \frac{250}{125}$$

$X = \textbf{2 mL}$

$$125 \overline{)250} \quad \substack{2 \\ -250 \\ \hline 0}$$

10. **Select label A.**

$$\frac{25 \text{ mg}}{5 \text{ mL}} = \frac{10 \text{ mg}}{X \text{ mL}}$$

$25X = 50$

$$\frac{25X}{25} = \frac{50}{25}$$

$X = \textbf{2 mL}$

11.　$\frac{0.05 \text{ mg}}{1 \text{ mL}} = \frac{0.25 \text{ mg}}{X \text{ mL}}$

$0.05X = 0.25$

$$\frac{0.05X}{0.05} = \frac{0.25}{0.05}$$

$X = \textbf{5 mL}$

$$0.05 \overline{)0.25} \quad \substack{5 \\ -25 \\ \hline 0}$$

12.　$\frac{10 \text{ g}}{15 \text{ mL}} = \frac{20 \text{ g}}{X \text{ mL}}$

$10X = 300$

$$\frac{10X}{10} = \frac{300}{10}$$

$X = \textbf{30 mL}$

13.　$\frac{10 \text{ mL}}{1 \text{ dose}} = \frac{473 \text{ mL}}{X \text{ doses}}$

$10X = 473$

$$\frac{10X}{10} = \frac{473}{10}$$

$X = \textbf{47.3 or 47 full doses}$

$473 \div 10 = 47.3$

14.　$\frac{2.5 \text{ mg}}{5 \text{ mL}} = \frac{2.5 \text{ mg}}{X \text{ mL}}$

$2.5X = 12.5$

$$\frac{2.5X}{2.5} = \frac{12.5}{2.5}$$

$X = \textbf{5 mL}$

$$2.5 \overline{)12.5} \quad \substack{5 \\ -125 \\ \hline 0}$$

15. 30 mL ordered per administration,

　　30 mL unit dose available.

　　30 min p.c. and h.s = 4 administrations per day.

　　4 containers are needed for a 24-hour period,

　　p.c. administration times are **0900, 1300, 1900.**

Practice Problems—Chapter 7 (page 123)

1. $\dfrac{1 \text{ g}}{1000 \text{ mg}} = \dfrac{0.5 \text{ g}}{\text{X mg}}$

$$X = 0.5 \times 1000 = 500 \text{ mg}$$

$$\dfrac{500 \text{ mg}}{\text{tab}} = \dfrac{250 \text{ mg}}{\text{X tab}}$$

$$500X = 250$$

$$\dfrac{500X}{500} = \dfrac{25\cancel{0}}{50\cancel{0}}$$

$$X = \dfrac{1}{2} \text{ tablet}$$

2. $\dfrac{\text{gr i}}{60 \text{ mg}} = \dfrac{\text{gr ss}}{\text{X mg}}$

$$X = \dfrac{1}{2} \times 60 = 30 \text{ mg}$$

$$\dfrac{15 \text{ mg}}{1 \text{ tab}} = \dfrac{30 \text{ mg}}{\text{X tab}}$$

$$15X = 30$$

$$\dfrac{15X}{15} = \dfrac{30}{15}$$

$$X = \mathbf{2 \text{ tablets}}$$

3. $\dfrac{1 \text{ mg}}{1000 \text{ mcg}} = \dfrac{0.075 \text{ mg}}{\text{X mcg}}$

$$X = 0.075 \times 1000 = 75 \text{ mcg}$$

$$\dfrac{150 \text{ mcg}}{1 \text{ tab}} = \dfrac{75 \text{ mcg}}{\text{X tab}}$$

$$150X = 75$$

$$\dfrac{150X}{150} = \dfrac{75}{150}$$

$$X = \dfrac{1}{2} \text{ tablet}$$

4. $\dfrac{\text{gr i}}{60 \text{ mg}} = \dfrac{\text{gr } \frac{1}{6}}{\text{X mg}}$

$$X = \dfrac{1}{6} \times 60 = 10 \text{ mg}$$

$$\dfrac{20 \text{ mg}}{5 \text{ mL}} = \dfrac{10 \text{ mg}}{\text{X mL}}$$

$$20X = 50$$

$$\dfrac{20X}{20} = \dfrac{5\cancel{0}}{2\cancel{0}}$$

$$X = \dfrac{5}{2} = \mathbf{2.5 \text{ mL}}$$

5. $\dfrac{250 \text{ mg}}{5 \text{ mL}} = \dfrac{500 \text{ mg}}{\text{X mL}}$

$$250X = 2500$$

$$\dfrac{250X}{250} = \dfrac{250\cancel{0}}{25\cancel{0}}$$

$$X = \mathbf{10 \text{ mL}}$$

6. $\dfrac{10 \text{ mg}}{1 \text{ tab}} = \dfrac{20 \text{ mg}}{\text{X tab}}$

$$10X = 20$$

$$\dfrac{10X}{10} = \dfrac{20}{10}$$

$$X = \mathbf{2 \text{ tablets}}$$

7. $\dfrac{250 \text{ mg}}{5 \text{ mL}} = \dfrac{500 \text{ mg}}{\text{X mL}}$

$$250X = 2500$$

$$\dfrac{250X}{250} = \dfrac{2500}{250}$$

$$X = \mathbf{10 \text{ mL}}$$

8. $\dfrac{1 \text{ g}}{1000 \text{ mg}} = \dfrac{0.1 \text{ g}}{\text{X mg}}$

$$X = 0.1 \times 1000 = 100 \text{ mg}$$

$$\dfrac{100 \text{ mg}}{1 \text{ tab}} = \dfrac{150 \text{ mg}}{\text{X tab}}$$

$$100X = 150$$

$$\dfrac{100X}{100} = \dfrac{15\cancel{0}}{10\cancel{0}}$$

$$X = \mathbf{1\dfrac{1}{2} \text{ tablets}}$$

9. $\dfrac{\text{gr i}}{60 \text{ mg}} = \dfrac{\text{gr } \frac{3}{4}}{\text{X mg}}$

$$X = \dfrac{3}{\cancel{4}} \times \overset{15}{\cancel{60}} = 45 \text{ mg}$$

$$\dfrac{30 \text{ mg}}{1 \text{ tab}} = \dfrac{45 \text{ mg}}{\text{X tab}}$$

$$30X = 45$$

$$\dfrac{30X}{30} = \dfrac{45}{30} = \dfrac{3}{2}$$

$$X = \mathbf{1\dfrac{1}{2} \text{ tablets}}$$

10. $\dfrac{\text{gr i}}{60 \text{ mg}} = \dfrac{\text{gr } \frac{1}{4}}{\text{X mg}}$

$$X = \dfrac{3}{\cancel{4}} \times \overset{15}{\cancel{60}}$$

$$X = 15 \text{ mg}$$

$$\dfrac{30 \text{ mg}}{1 \text{ tab}} = \dfrac{15 \text{ mg}}{\text{X tab}}$$

$$30X = 15$$

$$\dfrac{30X}{30} = \dfrac{15}{30}$$

$$X = \dfrac{1}{2} \text{ tablet}$$

11. $\dfrac{20 \text{ mg}}{1 \text{ tab}} = \dfrac{30 \text{ mg}}{\text{X tab}}$

$$20X = 30$$

$$\dfrac{20X}{20} = \dfrac{30}{20}$$

$$X = \mathbf{1\dfrac{1}{2} \text{ tablets}}$$

12. $\dfrac{1 \text{ mg}}{1000 \text{ mcg}} = \dfrac{0.3 \text{ mg}}{X \text{ mcg}}$

$X = 0.3 \times 1000$

$X = 300 \text{ mcg}$

$\dfrac{300 \text{ mcg}}{1 \text{ tab}} = \dfrac{300 \text{ mcg}}{X \text{ tab}}$

$300X = 300$

$\dfrac{300X}{300} = \dfrac{300}{300}$

$X = \textbf{1 tablet}$

13. $\dfrac{40 \text{ mg}}{1 \text{ tab}} = \dfrac{60 \text{ mg}}{X \text{ tab}}$

$40X = 60$

$\dfrac{40X}{40} = \dfrac{60}{40}$

$X = \mathbf{1\frac{1}{2}}$ **tablets**

14. $\dfrac{\text{gr i}}{60 \text{ mg}} = \dfrac{\text{gr } \frac{1}{8}}{X \text{ mg}}$

$X = \dfrac{1}{\underset{2}{\cancel{8}}} \times \overset{15}{\cancel{60}} = \dfrac{15}{2}$

$X = 7.5 \text{ mg}$

$\dfrac{7.5 \text{ mg}}{1 \text{ tab}} = \dfrac{7.5 \text{ mg}}{X \text{ tab}}$

$7.5X = 7.5$

$\dfrac{7.5X}{7.5} = \dfrac{7.5}{7.5}$

$X = \textbf{1 tablet}$

15. $\dfrac{400,000 \text{ U}}{1 \text{ tab}} = \dfrac{400,000 \text{ U}}{X \text{ tab}}$

$400,000X = 400,000$

$\dfrac{400,000X}{400,000} = \dfrac{400,000}{400,000}$

$X = \textbf{1 tablet}$

16. **Select 5 mg tablets.**

$\dfrac{5 \text{ mg}}{1 \text{ tab}} = \dfrac{7.5 \text{ mg}}{X \text{ tab}}$

$5X = 7.5$

$\dfrac{5X}{5} = \dfrac{7.5}{5}$

$X = \mathbf{1\frac{1}{2}}$ **tablets**

$$5 \overline{\smash{)}7.5} \quad \begin{array}{r} 1.5 \\ \hline \end{array}$$
$$\begin{array}{r} 1.5 \\ 5{\overline{\smash{)}7.5}} \\ -5 \\ \hline 25 \\ -25 \\ \hline 0 \end{array}$$

17. $\dfrac{200,000 \text{ U}}{5 \text{ mL}} = \dfrac{300,000 \text{ U}}{X \text{ mL}}$

$200,000X = 1,500,000$

$\dfrac{200,000X}{200,000} = \dfrac{1,500,000}{200,000}$

$X = \textbf{7.5 mL or } \mathbf{\frac{1}{2}}$ **t**

18. $\dfrac{1 \text{ g}}{1000 \text{ mg}} = \dfrac{0.75 \text{ g}}{X \text{ mg}}$

$X = 0.75 \times 1000$

$X = 750 \text{ mg}$

$\dfrac{500 \text{ mg}}{1 \text{ tab}} = \dfrac{750 \text{ mg}}{X \text{ tab}}$

$500X = 750$

$\dfrac{500X}{500} = \dfrac{750}{500}$

$X = \mathbf{1\frac{1}{2}}$ **tablets**

19. $\dfrac{0.125 \text{ mg}}{1 \text{ tab}} = \dfrac{0.25 \text{ mg}}{X \text{ tab}}$

$0.125X = 0.25$

$\dfrac{0.125X}{0.125} = \dfrac{0.25}{0.125}$

$X = \textbf{2 tablets}$

$$\begin{array}{r} 2 \\ 0.125{\overline{\smash{)}0.250}} \\ -250 \\ \hline 0 \end{array}$$

20. $\text{gr i} = 60 \text{ mg}$

$\dfrac{30 \text{ mg}}{1 \text{ cap}} = \dfrac{60 \text{ mg}}{X \text{ cap}}$

$30X = 60$

$\dfrac{30X}{30} = \dfrac{60}{30}$

$X = \textbf{2 capsules}$

21. $\dfrac{1 \text{ mg}}{1000 \text{ mcg}} = \dfrac{0.75 \text{ mg}}{X \text{ mcg}}$

$X = 0.75 \times 1000$

$X = 750 \text{ mcg}$

Select 0.75 mg tablets.

$\dfrac{750 \text{ mcg}}{1 \text{ tab}} = \dfrac{750 \text{ mcg}}{X \text{ tab}}$

$750X = 750$

$\dfrac{750X}{750} = \dfrac{750}{750}$

$X = \textbf{1 tablet}$

22. $\dfrac{25 \text{ mg}}{1 \text{ tab}} = \dfrac{12.5 \text{ mg}}{X \text{ tab}}$

$25X = 12.5$

$\dfrac{25X}{25} = \dfrac{12.5}{25}$

$X = \mathbf{\frac{1}{2}}$ **tablet**

$$\begin{array}{r} 0.5 \\ 25{\overline{\smash{)}12.5}} \\ -125 \\ \hline 0 \end{array}$$

23. $\dfrac{25 \text{ mg}}{1 \text{ tab}} = \dfrac{50 \text{ mg}}{X \text{ tab}}$

$25X = 50$

$\dfrac{25X}{25} = \dfrac{50}{25}$

$X = \textbf{2 tablets}$

24. $\dfrac{1\text{ g}}{1000\text{ mg}} = \dfrac{1.5\text{ g}}{X\text{ mg}}$

$X = 1.5 \times 1000$

$X = 1500\text{ mg}$

$\dfrac{750\text{ mg}}{1\text{ tab}} = \dfrac{1500\text{ mg}}{X\text{ tab}}$

$750X = 1500$

$\dfrac{750X}{750} = \dfrac{1500}{750}$

$X = \textbf{2 tablets}$

25. $1\text{ g} = 1000\text{ mg}$

$\dfrac{500\text{ mg}}{1\text{ tab}} = \dfrac{1000\text{ mg}}{X\text{ tab}}$

$500X = 1000$

$\dfrac{500X}{500} = \dfrac{1000}{500}$

$X = \textbf{2 tablets}$

26. **Select label D.**

$\dfrac{200\text{ mg}}{1\text{ tab}} = \dfrac{200\text{ mg}}{X\text{ tab}}$

$200X = 200$

$\dfrac{200X}{200} = \dfrac{200}{200}$

$X = \textbf{1 tablet}$

27. **Select label A.**

$\dfrac{60\text{ mg}}{1\text{ tab}} = \dfrac{60\text{ mg}}{X\text{ tab}}$

$60X = 60$

$\dfrac{60X}{60} = \dfrac{60}{60}$

$X = \textbf{1 tablet}$

28. **Select label C.**

$\dfrac{1\text{ mg}}{1000\text{ mcg}} = \dfrac{0.125\text{ mg}}{X\text{ mcg}}$

$X = 0.125 \times 1000$

$X = 125\text{ mcg}$

$\dfrac{125\text{ mcg}}{1\text{ tab}} = \dfrac{125\text{ mcg}}{X\text{ tab}}$

$125X = 125$

$\dfrac{125X}{125} = \dfrac{125}{125}$

$X = \textbf{1 tablet}$

29. **Select label B.**

$\dfrac{75\text{ mg}}{1\text{ tab}} = \dfrac{150\text{ mg}}{X\text{ tab}}$

$75X = 150$

$\dfrac{75X}{75} = \dfrac{150}{75}$

$X = \textbf{2 tablets}$

30. **Select label J.**

$\dfrac{0.1\text{ mg}}{1\text{ tab}} = \dfrac{0.2\text{ mg}}{X\text{ tab}}$

$0.1X = 0.2$

$\dfrac{0.1X}{0.1} = \dfrac{0.2}{0.1}$

$X = \textbf{2 tablets}$

31. **Select label G.**

$\dfrac{5\text{ mg}}{\text{tab}} = \dfrac{10\text{ mg}}{X\text{ tab}}$

$5X = 10$

$\dfrac{5X}{5} = \dfrac{10}{5}$

$X = \textbf{2 tablets}$

32. **Select label F.**

$\dfrac{250\text{ mg}}{5\text{ mL}} = \dfrac{250\text{ mg}}{X\text{ mL}}$

$250X = 1250$

$\dfrac{250X}{250} = \dfrac{1250}{250}$

$X = \textbf{5 mL}$

33. **Select label H.**

$\dfrac{15\text{ mg}}{1\text{ tab}} = \dfrac{30\text{ mg}}{X\text{ tab}}$

$15X = 30$

$\dfrac{15X}{15} = \dfrac{30}{15}$

$X = \textbf{2 tablets}$

34. **Select label E.**

$\dfrac{20\text{ mEq}}{15\text{ mL}} = \dfrac{40\text{ mEq}}{X\text{ mL}}$

$20X = 600$

$\dfrac{20X}{20} = \dfrac{600}{20}$

$X = \textbf{30 mL}$

35. **Select label M.**

$\dfrac{2.5\text{ mg}}{1\text{ cap}} = \dfrac{5\text{ mg}}{X\text{ cap}}$

$2.5X = 5$

$\dfrac{2.5X}{2.5} = \dfrac{5}{2.5}$

$X = \textbf{2 capsules}$

36. **Select label N.**

$$\frac{\text{gr i}}{60 \text{ mg}} = \frac{\text{gr}}{\text{X mg}}$$

$$\frac{1}{60} = \frac{10}{\text{X}}$$

$$\text{X} = 600 \text{ mg}$$

$$\frac{600 \text{ mg}}{1 \text{ tab}} = \frac{600 \text{ mg}}{\text{X tab}}$$

$$600\text{X} = 600$$

$$\frac{600\text{X}}{600} = \frac{600}{600}$$

$$\text{X} = \textbf{1 tablet}$$

37. **Select label L.**

$$\frac{1 \text{ g}}{1000 \text{ mg}} = \frac{0.6 \text{ g}}{\text{X mg}}$$

$$\text{X} = 0.6 \times 1000$$

$$\text{X} = 600 \text{ mg}$$

$$\frac{300 \text{ mg}}{1 \text{ cap}} = \frac{600 \text{ mg}}{\text{X cap}}$$

$$300\text{X} = 600$$

$$\frac{300\text{X}}{300} = \frac{600}{300}$$

$$\text{X} = \textbf{2 capsules}$$

38. **Select label K.**

$$\frac{40 \text{ mg}}{1 \text{ tab}} = \frac{40 \text{ mg}}{\text{X tab}}$$

$$40\text{X} = 40$$

$$\frac{40\text{X}}{40} = \frac{40}{40}$$

$$\text{X} = \textbf{1 tablet}$$

39. **Select label O.**

$$\frac{100 \text{ mg}}{1 \text{ tab}} = \frac{100 \text{ mg}}{\text{X tab}}$$

$$100\text{X} = 100$$

$$\frac{100\text{X}}{100} = \frac{100}{100}$$

$$\text{X} = \textbf{1 tablet}$$

40. **Select label P.**

Order reads:

Give **1 tablet** of Darvocet-N 100

41. **Select label B.**

$$\frac{400 \text{ mg}}{1 \text{ tab}} = \frac{400 \text{ mg}}{\text{X tab}}$$

$$400\text{X} = 400$$

$$\frac{400\text{X}}{400} = \frac{400}{400}$$

$$\text{X} = \textbf{1 tablet}$$

42. $$\frac{80 \text{ mg}}{1 \text{ tab}} = \frac{80 \text{ mg}}{\text{X tab}}$$

$$80\text{X} = 80$$

$$\frac{80\text{X}}{80} = \frac{80}{80}$$

$$\text{X} = \textbf{1 tablet}$$

43. **Select label A.**

$$\frac{20 \text{ mg}}{1 \text{ tab}} = \frac{20 \text{ mg}}{\text{X tab}}$$

$$20\text{X} = 20$$

$$\frac{20\text{X}}{20} = \frac{20}{20}$$

$$\text{X} = \textbf{1 tablet}$$

44. $$\frac{600 \text{ mg}}{1 \text{ tab}} = \frac{600 \text{ mg}}{\text{X tab}}$$

$$600\text{X} = 600$$

$$\frac{600\text{X}}{600} = \frac{600}{600}$$

$$\text{X} = \textbf{1 tablet}$$

45. **Select label B.**

$$\frac{50 \text{ mg}}{1 \text{ mL}} = \frac{50 \text{ mg}}{\text{X mL}}$$

$$50\text{X} = 50$$

$$\frac{50\text{X}}{50} = \frac{50}{50}$$

$$\text{X} = \textbf{1 mL}$$

Review Set 23 (page 139)

1. (gr i = 60 mg)

$$\frac{\text{gr i}}{60 \text{ mg}} = \frac{\text{gr} \frac{1}{4}}{\text{X mg}}$$

$$X = \frac{1}{\cancel{4}} \times \overset{15}{\cancel{60}}$$

$$X = 15 \text{ mg}$$

$$\frac{30 \text{ mg}}{1 \text{ mL}} = \frac{15 \text{ mg}}{\text{X mL}}$$

$$30X = 15$$

$$\frac{30X}{30} = \frac{15}{30}$$

$$X = \frac{1}{2} = \textbf{0.5 mL}$$

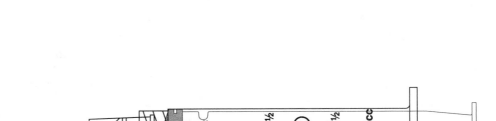

↑ 0.5 mL

2. $$\frac{600,000 \text{ U}}{1 \text{ mL}} = \frac{2,400,000 \text{ U}}{\text{X mL}}$$

$$600,000X = 2,400,000$$

$$\frac{600,000X}{600,000} = \frac{2,400,000}{600,000}$$

$$X = \textbf{4 mL}$$

**Divide the dosages into two injections
of 2.0 mL each.**

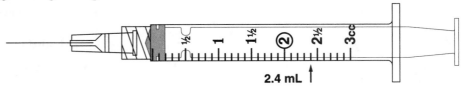

**2 mL in two syringes ↑
(4 mL total)**

3. No conversion necessary. Label gives mcg and mg.

$$\frac{500 \text{ mcg}}{2 \text{ mL}} = \frac{600 \text{ mcg}}{\text{X mL}}$$

$$500X = 1200$$

$$\frac{500X}{500} = \frac{1200}{500}$$

$$X = 2\frac{2}{5} = \textbf{2.4 mL}$$

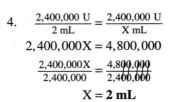

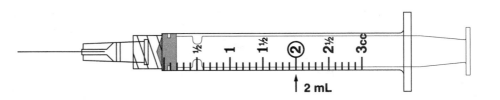

2.4 mL ↑

4. $$\frac{2,400,000 \text{ U}}{2 \text{ mL}} = \frac{2,400,000 \text{ U}}{\text{X mL}}$$

$$2,400,000X = 4,800,000$$

$$\frac{2,400,000X}{2,400,000} = \frac{4,800,000}{2,400,000}$$

$$X = \textbf{2 mL}$$

↑ 2 mL

5. $\dfrac{100 \text{ mg}}{1 \text{ mL}} = \dfrac{200 \text{ mg}}{X \text{ mL}}$

$100X = 200$

$\dfrac{100X}{100} = \dfrac{200}{100}$

$X = \textbf{2 mL stat dose}$

$\dfrac{100 \text{ mg}}{1 \text{ mL}} = \dfrac{100 \text{ mg}}{X \text{ mL}}$

$100X = 100$

$\dfrac{100X}{100} = \dfrac{100}{100}$

$X = \textbf{1 mL q.6h dose}$

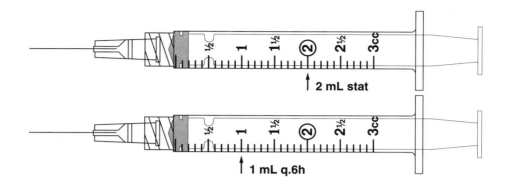

2 mL stat

1 mL q.6h

6. $\dfrac{10{,}000 \text{ U}}{1 \text{ mL}} = \dfrac{8{,}000 \text{ U}}{X \text{ mL}}$

$10{,}000X = 8000$

$\dfrac{10{,}000X}{10{,}000} = \dfrac{8000}{10{,}000}$

$X = \textbf{0.8 mL}$

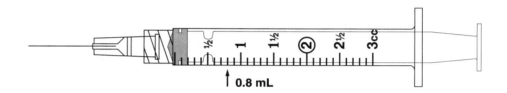

0.8 mL

7. $\dfrac{2 \text{ mEq}}{1 \text{ mL}} = \dfrac{15 \text{ mEq}}{X \text{ mL}}$

$2X = 15$

$\dfrac{2X}{2} = \dfrac{15}{2}$

$X = 7\dfrac{1}{2} = \textbf{7.5 mL}$

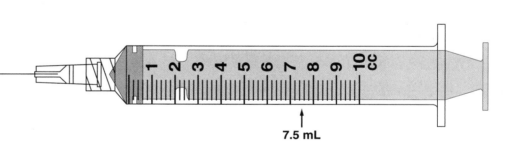

7.5 mL

8. $\dfrac{75 \text{ mg}}{1.5 \text{ mL}} = \dfrac{60 \text{ mg}}{X \text{ mL}}$

$75X = 90$

$\dfrac{75X}{75} = \dfrac{90}{75}$

$X = \textbf{1.2 mL}$

$\begin{array}{r} 60 \\ \times 1.5 \\ \hline 300 \\ 60 \\ \hline 90.0 \end{array}$

$\begin{array}{r} 1.2 \\ 75 \overline{) 90.0} \\ -75 \\ \hline 150 \\ -150 \\ \hline 0 \end{array}$

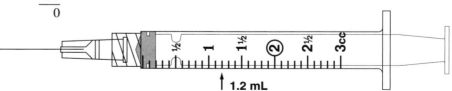

1.2 mL

9. (gr i = 60 mg)

$$\frac{\text{gr i}}{60 \text{ mg}} = \frac{\text{gr} \frac{1}{100}}{\text{X mg}}$$

$$X = \frac{1}{10\cancel{0}} \times 6\cancel{0}$$

$$X = 0.6 \text{ mg}$$

$$\frac{0.4 \text{ mg}}{1 \text{ mL}} = \frac{0.6 \text{ mg}}{\text{X mL}}$$

$$0.4X = 0.6$$

$$\frac{0.4X}{0.4} = \frac{0.6}{0.4}$$

$$X = \textbf{1.5 mL}$$

$$\begin{array}{r} 1.5 \\ 0.4\overline{)0.6.0} \\ \underline{-4} \\ 20 \\ 20 \end{array}$$

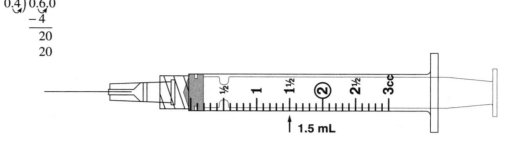

↑ **1.5 mL**

10. (gr i = 60 mg)

$$\frac{\text{gr i}}{60 \text{ mg}} = \frac{\text{gr} \frac{1}{6}}{\text{X mg}}$$

$$X = \frac{1}{\cancel{6}} \times \overset{10}{\cancel{60}}$$

$$X = 10 \text{ mg}$$

$$\frac{10 \text{ mg}}{1 \text{ mL}} = \frac{10 \text{ mg}}{\text{X mL}}$$

$$10X = 10$$

$$\frac{10X}{10} = \frac{10}{10}$$

$$X = \textbf{1 mL}$$

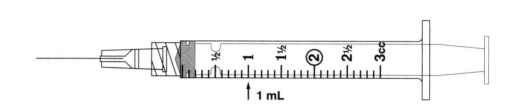

↑ **1 mL**

11. $$\frac{300{,}000 \text{ U}}{1 \text{ mL}} = \frac{400{,}000 \text{ U}}{\text{X mL}}$$

$$300{,}000X = 400{,}000$$

$$\frac{300{,}000X}{300{,}000} = \frac{400{,}000}{300{,}000}$$

$$X = \frac{4}{3} = \textbf{1.3 mL}$$

$$\begin{array}{r} 1.33 \\ 3\overline{)4.00} \\ \underline{-3} \\ 10 \\ \underline{-9} \\ 10 \\ \underline{-9} \\ 1 \end{array}$$

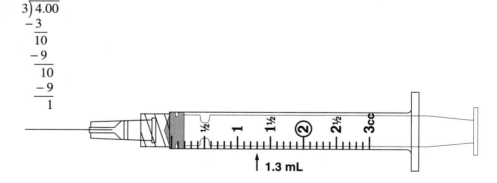

↑ **1.3 mL**

12. $$\frac{10{,}000 \text{ U}}{1 \text{ mL}} = \frac{4500 \text{ U}}{\text{X mL}}$$

$$10{,}000X = 4500$$

$$\frac{10{,}000X}{10{,}000} = \frac{4500}{10{,}000}$$

$$X = \textbf{0.45 mL}$$

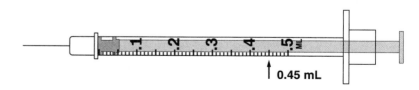

↑ **0.45 mL**

13. $$\frac{5 \text{ mg}}{1 \text{ mL}} = \frac{7.5 \text{ mg}}{\text{X mL}}$$

$$5X = 7.5$$

$$\frac{5X}{5} = \frac{7.5}{5}$$

$$X = \textbf{1.5 mL}$$

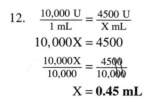

$$\begin{array}{r} 1.5 \\ 5\overline{)7.5} \\ \underline{-5} \\ 25 \\ \underline{-25} \\ 0 \end{array}$$

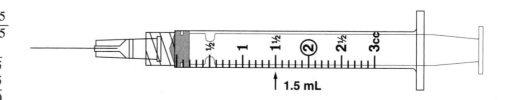

↑ **1.5 mL**

14. $\dfrac{25 \text{ mg}}{1 \text{ mL}} = \dfrac{20 \text{ mg}}{X \text{ mL}}$

$25X = 20$

$\dfrac{25X}{25} = \dfrac{20}{25}$

$X = \dfrac{4}{5} = \mathbf{0.8 \ mL}$

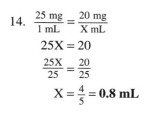

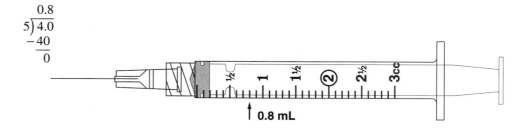

↑ 0.8 mL

15. $\dfrac{40 \text{ mg}}{1 \text{ cc}} = \dfrac{60 \text{ mg}}{X \text{ cc}}$

$40X = 60$

$\dfrac{40X}{40} = \dfrac{60}{40}$

$X = \dfrac{3}{2} = \mathbf{1.5 \ cc}$

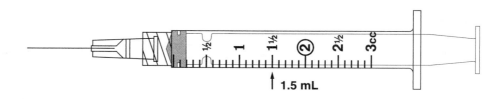

↑ 1.5 mL

16. $\dfrac{2 \text{ mg}}{1 \text{ mL}} = \dfrac{3 \text{ mg}}{X \text{ mL}}$

$2X = 3$

$\dfrac{2X}{2} = \dfrac{3}{2}$

$X = \mathbf{1.5 \ mL}$

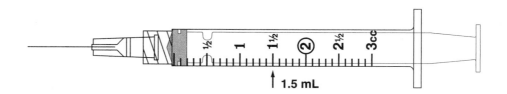

↑ 1.5 mL

17. $\dfrac{1 \text{ mg}}{1 \text{ mL}} = \dfrac{0.5 \text{ mg}}{X \text{ mL}}$

$X = \mathbf{0.5 \ mL}$

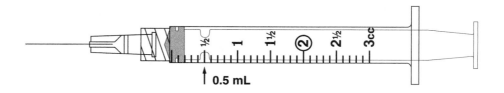

↑ 0.5 mL

18. $\dfrac{25 \text{ mg}}{1 \text{ mL}} = \dfrac{20 \text{ mg}}{X \text{ mL}}$

$25X = 20$

$\dfrac{25X}{25} = \dfrac{20}{25}$

$X = \dfrac{4}{5} = \mathbf{0.8 \ mL}$

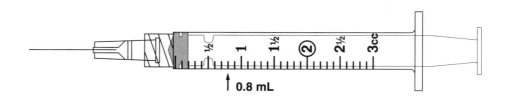

↑ 0.8 mL

19. $\dfrac{50 \text{ mg}}{1 \text{ mL}} = \dfrac{12.5 \text{ mg}}{X \text{ mL}}$

$50X = 12.5$

$\dfrac{50X}{50} = \dfrac{12.5}{50}$

$X = \mathbf{0.25 \ mL}$

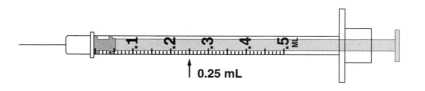

↑ 0.25 mL

20. $\dfrac{10 \text{ mg}}{2 \text{ mL}} = \dfrac{8 \text{ mg}}{X \text{ mL}}$

$10X = 16$

$\dfrac{10X}{10} = \dfrac{16}{10}$

$X = \mathbf{1.6 \ mL}$

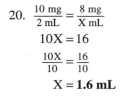

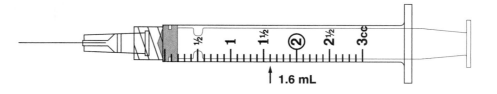

↑ 1.6 mL

Review Set 24 (page 147)

1. $\dfrac{280\ mg}{1\ mL} = \dfrac{250\ mg}{X\ mL}$

    $280X = 250$

    $\dfrac{280X}{280} = \dfrac{250}{280}$

    $\quad X = \mathbf{0.89\ mL}$

$$
\begin{array}{r}
0.892 \\
28\overline{)25.000} \\
-224 \\
\hline
260 \\
-252 \\
\hline
80 \\
-56 \\
\hline
24 \\
\end{array}
$$

Reconstitute with 1.5 mL and give 0.89 mL.

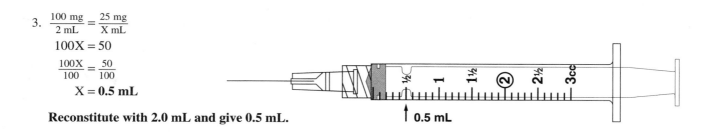

↑ 0.89 mL

2. $\quad 1\ g = 1000\ mg$

    $\dfrac{1000\ mg}{3\ mL} = \dfrac{500\ mg}{X\ mL}$

    $1000X = 1500$

    $\dfrac{1000X}{1000} = \dfrac{1500}{1000}$

    $\quad\quad X = \mathbf{1.5\ mL}$

Reconstitute with 5.0 mL and give 1.5 mL.

↑ 1.5 mL

3. $\dfrac{100\ mg}{2\ mL} = \dfrac{25\ mg}{X\ mL}$

    $100X = 50$

    $\dfrac{100X}{100} = \dfrac{50}{100}$

    $\quad X = \mathbf{0.5\ mL}$

Reconstitute with 2.0 mL and give 0.5 mL.

↑ 0.5 mL

4. $\quad 1\ g = 1000\ mg$

    $\dfrac{1000\ mg}{50\ mL} = \dfrac{250\ mg}{X\ mL}$

    $1000X = 12500$

    $\dfrac{1000X}{1000} = \dfrac{12500}{1000}$

    $\quad\quad X = \mathbf{12.5\ mL}$

Reconstitute with 50 mL and give 12.5 mL.

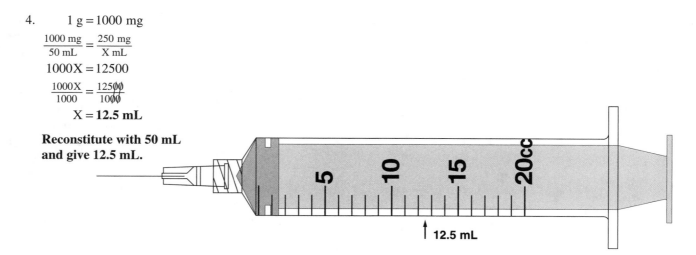

↑ 12.5 mL

5. $1\text{ g} = 1000\text{ mg}$

$$\frac{1000\text{ mg}}{50\text{ mL}} = \frac{300\text{ mg}}{X\text{ mL}}$$

$1000X = 15000$

$$\frac{1000X}{1000} = \frac{15000}{1000}$$

$X = \textbf{15 mL}$

Reconstitute with 50 mL and give 15 mL.

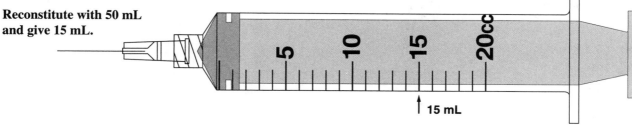

↑ **15 mL**

6. $\frac{250\text{ mg}}{1\text{ mL}} = \frac{500\text{ mg}}{X\text{ mL}}$

$250X = 500$

$\frac{250X}{250} = \frac{500}{250}$

$X = \textbf{2 mL}$

Reconstitute with 3.5 mL diluent and give 2 mL.

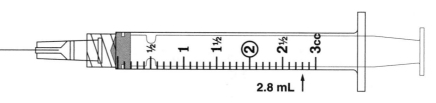

↑ **2 mL**

7. $\frac{62.5\text{ mg}}{1\text{ mL}} = \frac{175\text{ mg}}{X\text{ mL}}$

$62.5X = 175$

$\frac{62.5X}{62.5} = \frac{175}{62.5}$

$X = \textbf{2.8 mL}$

$$\begin{array}{r} 2.8 \\ 62.5\overline{)175.00} \\ -1250 \\ \hline 5000 \\ -5000 \\ \hline 0 \end{array}$$

Reconstitute with 8 mL and give 2.8 mL.

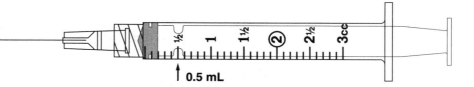

2.8 mL ↑

8. $1\text{ g} = 1000\text{ mg}$

$$\frac{1000\text{ mg}}{2.5\text{ mL}} = \frac{200\text{ mg}}{X\text{ mL}}$$

$1000X = 500$

$$\frac{1000X}{1000} = \frac{500}{1000}$$

$X = \textbf{0.5 mL}$

$$\begin{array}{r} 200 \\ \times 2.5 \\ \hline 1000 \\ 400 \\ \hline 500.0 \end{array}$$

Reconstitute with 4 mL diluent and give 0.5 mL.

↑ **0.5 mL**

9. $$\frac{500,000 \text{ U}}{1 \text{ mL}} = \frac{500,000 \text{ U}}{X \text{ mL}}$$

$$500,000X = 500,000$$

$$\frac{500,000X}{500,000} = \frac{500,000}{500,000}$$

$$X = \mathbf{1 \text{ mL}}$$

Reconstitute with 1.6 mL and give 1 mL.

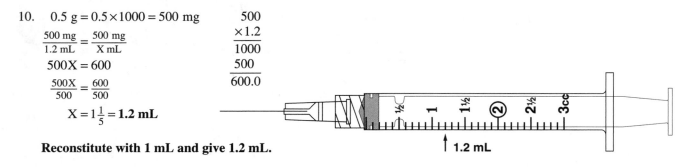
↑ 1 mL

10. $0.5 \text{ g} = 0.5 \times 1000 = 500 \text{ mg}$

$$\frac{500 \text{ mg}}{1.2 \text{ mL}} = \frac{500 \text{ mg}}{X \text{ mL}}$$

$$500X = 600$$

$$\frac{500X}{500} = \frac{600}{500}$$

$$X = 1\frac{1}{5} = \mathbf{1.2 \text{ mL}}$$

$$\begin{array}{r} 500 \\ \times 1.2 \\ \hline 1000 \\ 500 \\ \hline 600.0 \end{array}$$

Reconstitute with 1 mL and give 1.2 mL.

↑ 1.2 mL

11. $$\frac{500,000 \text{ U}}{1 \text{ mL}} = \frac{400,000 \text{ U}}{X \text{ mL}}$$

$$500,000X = 400,000$$

$$\frac{500,000X}{500,000} = \frac{400,000}{500,000}$$

$$X = \frac{4}{5} = \mathbf{0.8 \text{ mL}}$$

Reconstitute with 1.6 mL and give 0.8 mL.

↑ 0.8 mL

12. $$\frac{330 \text{ mg}}{1 \text{ mL}} = \frac{500 \text{ mg}}{X \text{ mL}}$$

$$330X = 500$$

$$\frac{330X}{330} = \frac{500}{330}$$

$$X = \mathbf{1.5 \text{ mL}}$$

$$\begin{array}{r} 1.51 \\ 33\overline{)50.00} \\ -33 \\ \hline 170 \\ -165 \\ \hline 50 \end{array}$$

**Reconstitute with 2.5 mL
and give 1.5 mL.**

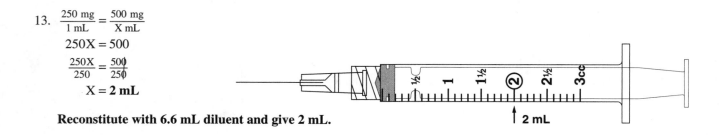
↑ 1.5 mL

13. $$\frac{250 \text{ mg}}{1 \text{ mL}} = \frac{500 \text{ mg}}{X \text{ mL}}$$

$$250X = 500$$

$$\frac{250X}{250} = \frac{500}{250}$$

$$X = \mathbf{2 \text{ mL}}$$

Reconstitute with 6.6 mL diluent and give 2 mL.

↑ 2 mL

14. $\dfrac{150\ U}{1\ mL} = \dfrac{75\ U}{X\ mL}$

$150X = 75$

$\dfrac{150X}{150} = \dfrac{75}{150}$

$X = \textbf{0.5 mL}$

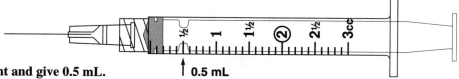

Reconstitute with 10 mL diluent and give 0.5 mL.

↑ **0.5 mL**

15. $\dfrac{225\ mg}{1\ mL} = \dfrac{250\ mg}{X\ mL}$

$225X = 250$

$\dfrac{225X}{225} = \dfrac{250}{225}$

$X = \textbf{1.1 mL}$

$$\begin{array}{r} 1.11 \\ 225\overline{)250.00} \\ -\,225 \\ \hline 250 \\ -\,225 \\ \hline 250 \end{array}$$

**Reconstitute with 2 mL
and give 1.1 mL.**

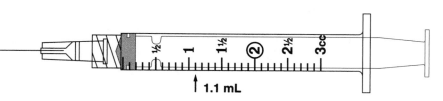

↑ **1.1 mL**

Review Set 25 (page 157)

1. **In a U-100 insulin syringe**

2. **Lo-Dose U-100 insulin syringe**

3. $\dfrac{100\ U}{1\ mL} = \dfrac{20\ U}{X\ mL}$

$100X = 20$

$\dfrac{100X}{100} = \dfrac{20}{100}$

$X = \textbf{0.2 mL}$

0.2 mL measured in a tuberculin syringe

4. $\dfrac{100\ U}{1\ mL} = \dfrac{60\ U}{X\ mL}$

$100X = 60$

$\dfrac{100X}{100} = \dfrac{60}{100}$

$X = \textbf{0.6 mL}$

5. $\dfrac{100\ U}{1\ mL} = \dfrac{25\ U}{X\ mL}$

$100X = 25$

$\dfrac{100X}{100} = \dfrac{25}{100}$

$X = \textbf{0.25 mL}$

6. **insulin**

7. **False**

8. **68 U**

9. **15 U**

10. **23 U**

11. **57 U**

12.
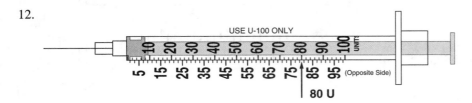

13.
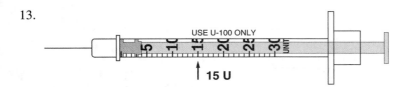

14.
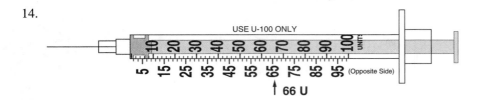

15.
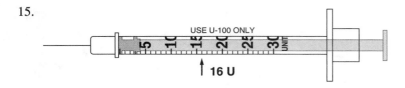

16.
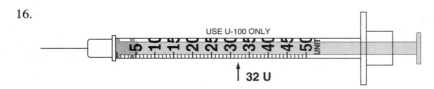

17.
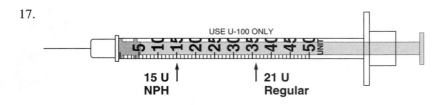

18.
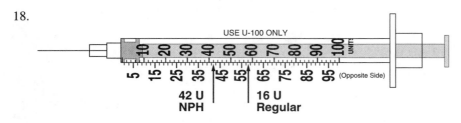

19.

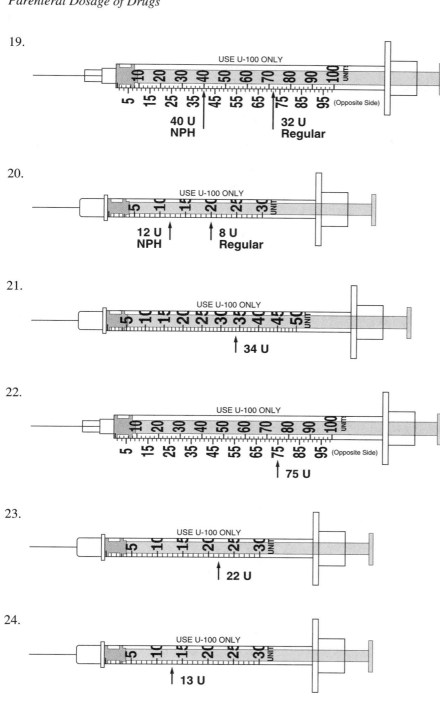

USE U-100 ONLY

40 U
NPH

32 U
Regular

(Opposite Side)

20.

USE U-100 ONLY

12 U
NPH

8 U
Regular

21.

USE U-100 ONLY

34 U

22.

USE U-100 ONLY

(Opposite Side)

75 U

23.

USE U-100 ONLY

22 U

24.

USE U-100 ONLY

13 U

25.

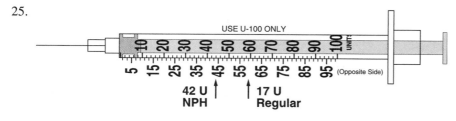

USE U-100 ONLY

(Opposite Side)

42 U
NPH

17 U
Regular

Review Set 26 (page 161)

1. 20% = 20 g in 100 mL

$$\frac{20 \text{ g}}{100 \text{ mL}} = \frac{4 \text{ g}}{X \text{ mL}}$$
$$20X = 400$$
$$\frac{20X}{20} = \frac{40\cancel{0}}{2\cancel{0}}$$
$$X = \textbf{20 mL}$$

2. $1:2000 = \frac{1 \text{ g}}{2000 \text{ mL}} = \frac{1000 \text{ mg}}{2000 \text{ mL}} = \frac{1 \text{ mg}}{2 \text{ mL}}$

$$\frac{1 \text{ mg}}{2 \text{ mL}} = \frac{0.5 \text{ mg}}{X \text{ mL}}$$
$$X = \textbf{1 mL}$$

3. $1:1000 = \frac{1 \text{ g}}{1000 \text{ mL}} = \frac{1000 \text{ mg}}{1000 \text{ mL}} = \frac{1 \text{ mg}}{1 \text{ mL}}$

$$\frac{1 \text{ mg}}{1 \text{ mL}} = \frac{0.3 \text{ mg}}{X \text{ mL}}$$
$$X = \textbf{0.3 mL}$$

4. $1:2000 = \frac{1 \text{ mg}}{2 \text{ mL}}$ (see #2)

$$\frac{1 \text{ mg}}{2 \text{ mL}} = \frac{0.25 \text{ mg}}{X \text{ mL}}$$
$$X = 0.25 \times 2$$
$$X = \textbf{0.5 mL}$$

5. $\frac{1 \text{ g}}{\text{gr } 15} = \frac{X \text{ g}}{\text{gr viiss}}$

$$\frac{1}{15} = \frac{X}{7.5}$$
$$15X = 7.5$$
$$\frac{15X}{15} = \frac{7.5}{15}$$
$$X = 0.5 \text{ g}$$
$$25\% = \frac{25 \text{ g}}{100 \text{ mL}} = \frac{1 \text{ g}}{4 \text{ mL}}$$
$$\frac{1 \text{ g}}{4 \text{ mL}} = \frac{0.5 \text{ g}}{X \text{ mL}}$$
$$X = 0.5 \times 4$$
$$X = \textbf{2 mL}$$

Practice Problems—Chapter 8 (page 165)

1. $\frac{50 \text{ mg}}{1 \text{ mL}} = \frac{20 \text{ mg}}{X \text{ mL}}$

$$50X = 20$$
$$\frac{50X}{50} = \frac{2\cancel{0}}{5\cancel{0}}$$
$$X = \textbf{0.4 mL}$$

Give 0.4 mL
Select 0.5 mL TB syringe

2. $\frac{\text{gr i}}{60 \text{ mg}} = \frac{\text{gr } \frac{1}{4}}{X \text{ mg}}$

$$X = \frac{1}{\cancel{4}} \times \cancel{60}^{\,15}$$
$${}^{1}$$
$$X = 15 \text{ mg}$$
$$\frac{15 \text{ mg}}{1 \text{ mL}} = \frac{15 \text{ mg}}{X \text{ mL}}$$
$$15X = 15$$
$$\frac{15X}{15} = \frac{15}{15}$$
$$X = \textbf{1 mL}$$

Give 1 mL
Select 3 cc syringe

3. Convert 0.6 mg to mcg.

1 mg = 1000 mcg

$$\frac{1 \text{ mg}}{1000 \text{ mcg}} = \frac{0.6 \text{ mg}}{X \text{ mcg}}$$
$$X = 0.6 \times 1000$$
$$X = 600 \text{ mcg}$$
$$\frac{500 \text{ mcg}}{2 \text{ mL}} = \frac{600 \text{ mcg}}{X \text{ mL}}$$
$$500X = 1200$$
$$\frac{500X}{500} = \frac{120\cancel{0}}{50\cancel{0}}$$
$$X = 2\frac{2}{5} = \textbf{2.4 mL}$$

Give 2.4 mL
Select 3 cc syringe

4. $\frac{25 \text{ mg}}{1 \text{ mL}} = \frac{15 \text{ mg}}{X \text{ mL}}$

$$25X = 15$$
$$\frac{25X}{25} = \frac{15}{25}$$
$$X = \frac{3}{5} = \textbf{0.6 mL}$$

Give 0.6 mL
Select 1 mL or 3 cc syringe

5. $\dfrac{250,000 \text{ U}}{1 \text{ mL}} = \dfrac{500,000 \text{ U}}{X \text{ mL}}$

$250,000X = 500,000$

$\dfrac{250,000X}{250,000} = \dfrac{500,000}{250,000}$

$X = \textbf{2 mL}$

Give 2 mL

Select 3 cc syringe

6. $0.6 \text{ g} = 0.6 \times 1000 = 600 \text{ mg}$

$\dfrac{600 \text{ mg}}{4 \text{ mL}} = \dfrac{300 \text{ mg}}{X \text{ mL}}$

$600X = 1200$

$\dfrac{600X}{600} = \dfrac{1200}{600}$

$X = \textbf{2 mL}$

Give 2 mL

Select 3 cc syringe

7. $\dfrac{1 \text{ mg}}{5 \text{ mL}} = \dfrac{3 \text{ mg}}{X \text{ mL}}$

$X = \textbf{15 mL}$

Give 15 mL

Select 20 cc syringe

8. $\dfrac{250 \text{ mg}}{1 \text{ mL}} = \dfrac{500 \text{ mg}}{X \text{ mL}}$

$250X = 500$

$\dfrac{250X}{250} = \dfrac{500}{250}$

$X = \textbf{2 mL}$

Give 2 mL

Select 3 cc syringe

9. $\dfrac{2 \text{ mEq}}{1 \text{ mL}} = \dfrac{30 \text{ mEq}}{X \text{ mL}}$

$2X = 30$

$\dfrac{2X}{2} = \dfrac{30}{2}$

$X = \textbf{15 mL}$

Give 15 mL

Select 20 cc syringe

10. $\dfrac{50 \text{ mg}}{1 \text{ mL}} = \dfrac{40 \text{ mg}}{X \text{ mL}}$

$50X = 40$

$\dfrac{50X}{50} = \dfrac{40}{50}$

$X = \dfrac{4}{5} = \textbf{0.8 mL}$

Give 0.8 mL

Select 1 mL or 3 cc syringe

11. $\dfrac{10 \text{ mg}}{2 \text{ mL}} = \dfrac{5 \text{ mg}}{X \text{ mL}}$

$10X = 10$

$\dfrac{10X}{10} = \dfrac{10}{10}$

$X = \textbf{1 mL}$

Give 1 mL

Select 3 cc syringe

12. $\dfrac{200 \text{ mg}}{2 \text{ mL}} = \dfrac{100 \text{ mg}}{X \text{ mL}}$

$200X = 200$

$\dfrac{200X}{200} = \dfrac{200}{200}$

$X = \textbf{1 mL}$

Give 1 mL

Select 3 cc syringe

13. $\dfrac{100 \text{ mg}}{2 \text{ mL}} = \dfrac{25 \text{ mg}}{X \text{ mL}}$

$100X = 50$

$\dfrac{100X}{100} = \dfrac{50}{100}$

$X = \dfrac{1}{2} = \textbf{0.5 mL}$

Give 0.5 mL

Select 1 mL TB or 3 cc syringe

14. Convert gr $\frac{1}{100}$ to mg.

$\dfrac{\text{gr i}}{60 \text{ mg}} = \dfrac{\text{gr } \frac{1}{100}}{X \text{ mg}}$

$X = 60 \times \dfrac{1}{100}$

$X = 0.6 \text{ mg}$

$\dfrac{0.4 \text{ mg}}{1 \text{ mL}} = \dfrac{0.6 \text{ mg}}{X \text{ mL}}$

$0.4X = 0.6$

$\dfrac{0.4X}{0.4} = \dfrac{0.6}{0.4}$

$X = \textbf{1.5 mL}$

Give 1.5 mL

Select 3 cc syringe

15. $\dfrac{10 \text{ mg}}{2 \text{ mL}} = \dfrac{3 \text{ mg}}{X \text{ mL}}$

$10X = 6$

$\dfrac{10X}{10} = \dfrac{6}{10}$

$X = \textbf{0.6 mL}$

Give 0.6 mL

Select 1 ml TB or 3 cc syringe

16. $\dfrac{10,000 \text{ U}}{1 \text{ mL}} = \dfrac{6000 \text{ U}}{X \text{ mL}}$

$10,000X = 6000$

$\dfrac{10,000X}{10,000} = \dfrac{6000}{10,000}$

$X = \textbf{0.6 mL}$

Give 0.6 mL

Select 1 mL TB or 3 cc syringe

17. $\dfrac{80 \text{ mg}}{2 \text{ mL}} = \dfrac{75 \text{ mg}}{X \text{ mL}}$

$80X = 150$

$\dfrac{80X}{80} = \dfrac{150}{80}$

$X = \textbf{1.9 mL}$

Give 1.9 mL

Select 3 cc syringe

$$\begin{array}{r} 1.87 \\ 8\overline{)15.00} \\ -8 \\ \hline 70 \\ -64 \\ \hline 60 \\ -56 \\ \hline 4 \end{array}$$

18. Convert gr $\dfrac{1}{10}$ to mg.

$\dfrac{\text{gr i}}{60 \text{ mg}} = \dfrac{\text{gr } \frac{1}{10}}{X \text{ mg}}$

$X = \dfrac{1}{1\cancel{0}} \times 6\cancel{0}$

$X = 6 \text{ mg}$

$\dfrac{10 \text{ mg}}{1 \text{ mL}} = \dfrac{6 \text{ mg}}{X \text{ mL}}$

$10X = 6$

$\dfrac{10X}{10} = \dfrac{6}{10}$

$X = \textbf{0.6 mL}$

Give 0.6 mL

Select 1 mL TB or 3 cc syringe

19. Convert gr $\dfrac{1}{150}$ to mg.

$\dfrac{\text{gr i}}{60 \text{ mg}} = \dfrac{\text{gr } \frac{1}{150}}{X \text{ mg}}$

$X = \dfrac{1}{15\cancel{0}} \times 6\cancel{0}$

$X = \dfrac{6}{15} = \dfrac{2}{5} = 0.4 \text{ mg}$

$\dfrac{0.4 \text{ mg}}{1 \text{ mL}} = \dfrac{0.4 \text{ mg}}{X \text{ mL}}$

$0.4X = 0.4$

$\dfrac{0.4X}{0.4} = \dfrac{0.4}{0.4}$

$X = \textbf{1 mL}$

Give 1 mL

Select 3 cc syringe

20. $\dfrac{100 \text{ mg}}{1 \text{ mL}} = \dfrac{120 \text{ mg}}{X \text{ mL}}$

$100X = 120$

$\dfrac{100X}{100} = \dfrac{120}{100}$

$X = \textbf{1.2 mL}$

Give 1.2 mL

Select 3 cc syringe

21. $\dfrac{330 \text{ mg}}{1 \text{ mL}} = \dfrac{500 \text{ mg}}{X \text{ mL}}$

$330X = 500$

$\dfrac{330X}{330} = \dfrac{500}{330}$

$X = \textbf{1.5 mL}$

Give 1.5 mL

Select 3 cc syringe

$$\begin{array}{r} 1.51 \\ 33\overline{)50.00} \\ -33 \\ \hline 170 \\ -165 \\ \hline 50 \\ -33 \\ \hline 17 \end{array}$$

22. $\dfrac{80 \text{ mg}}{2 \text{ mL}} = \dfrac{40 \text{ mg}}{X \text{ mL}}$

$80X = 80$

$\dfrac{80X}{80} = \dfrac{80}{80}$

$X = \textbf{1 mL}$

Give 1 mL

Select 3 cc syringe

23. $\dfrac{75 \text{ mg}}{1.5 \text{ mL}} = \dfrac{60 \text{ mg}}{X \text{ mL}}$

$75X = 90$

$\dfrac{75X}{75} = \dfrac{90}{75} = \dfrac{18}{15} = \dfrac{6}{5} = 1\dfrac{1}{5}$

$X = \textbf{1.2 mL}$

Give 1.2 mL

Select 3 cc syringe

24. $\dfrac{50 \text{ mg}}{1 \text{ mL}} = \dfrac{35 \text{ mg}}{X \text{ mL}}$

$50X = 35$

$\dfrac{50X}{50} = \dfrac{35}{50} = \dfrac{7}{10}$

$X = \textbf{0.7 mL}$

Give 0.7 mL

Select 1 mL or 3 cc syringe

25. Convert 0.75 mg to mcg.

1 mg = 1000 mcg

$\dfrac{1 \text{ mg}}{1000 \text{ mcg}} = \dfrac{0.75 \text{ mg}}{X \text{ mcg}}$

$X = 0.75 \times 1000$

$X = 750 \text{ mcg}$

$\dfrac{1000 \text{ mcg}}{1 \text{ mL}} = \dfrac{750 \text{ mcg}}{X \text{ mL}}$

$1000X = 750$

$\dfrac{1000X}{1000} = \dfrac{750}{1000}$

$X = \textbf{0.75 mL}$

Give 0.75 mL

Select 1 mL TB 3 cc syringe

26. $\dfrac{10 \text{ mg}}{1 \text{ mL}} = \dfrac{15 \text{ mg}}{X \text{ mL}}$

$10X = 15$

$\dfrac{10X}{10} = \dfrac{15}{10}$

$X = \textbf{1.5 mL}$

Give 1.5 mL

Select 3 cc syringe

27. $\dfrac{50 \text{ mg}}{1 \text{ mL}} = \dfrac{35 \text{ mg}}{X \text{ mL}}$

$50X = 35$

$\dfrac{50X}{50} = \dfrac{35}{50}$

$X = \dfrac{7}{10} = \textbf{0.7 mL}$

Give 0.7 mL

Select 1 mL TB or 3 cc syringe

28. $\dfrac{10{,}000 \text{ U}}{1 \text{ mL}} = \dfrac{8000 \text{ U}}{X \text{ mL}}$

$10{,}000X = 8000$

$\dfrac{10{,}000X}{10{,}000} = \dfrac{8000}{10{,}000}$

$X = \textbf{0.8 mL}$

Give 0.8 mL

Select 1 mL TB or 3 cc syringe

29. Convert gr $\frac{1}{10}$ to mg.

$\dfrac{\text{gr i}}{60 \text{ mg}} = \dfrac{\text{gr } \frac{1}{10}}{X \text{ mg}}$

$X = \dfrac{1}{10} \times 60$

$X = 6 \text{ mg}$

$\dfrac{6 \text{ mg}}{1 \text{ mL}} = \dfrac{6 \text{ mg}}{X \text{ mL}}$

$6X = 6$

$\dfrac{6X}{6} = \dfrac{6}{6}$

$X = \textbf{1 mL}$

Give 1 mL

Select 3 cc syringe

30. 1 g = 1000 mg

$\dfrac{1000 \text{ mg}}{5 \text{ mL}} = \dfrac{750 \text{ mg}}{X \text{ mL}}$

$1000X = 3750$

$\dfrac{1000X}{1000} = \dfrac{3750}{1000}$

$X = 3.75 = \textbf{3.8 mL}$

Give 3.8 mL

Select 5 cc syringe

31. $\dfrac{125 \text{ mg}}{1 \text{ mL}} = \dfrac{100 \text{ mg}}{X \text{ mL}}$

$125X = 100$

$\dfrac{125X}{125} = \dfrac{\overset{4}{100}}{\underset{5}{125}}$

$X = \dfrac{4}{5} = \textbf{0.8 mL}$

Give 0.8 mL

Select 1 mL TB or 3 cc syringe

32. Convert 0.4 mg to mcg.

$\dfrac{1 \text{ mg}}{1000 \text{ mcg}} = \dfrac{0.4 \text{ mg}}{X \text{ mcg}}$

$X = 0.4 \times 1000$

$X = 400 \text{ mcg}$

$\dfrac{500 \text{ mcg}}{2 \text{ mL}} = \dfrac{400 \text{ mcg}}{X \text{ mL}}$

$500X = 800$

$\dfrac{500X}{500} = \dfrac{800}{500}$

$X = \dfrac{8}{5} = 1\dfrac{3}{5} = \textbf{1.6 mL}$

Give 1.6 mL

Select 3 cc syringe

33. $\dfrac{20 \text{ mg}}{2 \text{ mL}} = \dfrac{60 \text{ mg}}{X \text{ mL}}$

$20X = 120$

$\dfrac{20X}{20} = \dfrac{12\cancel{0}}{2\cancel{0}}$

$X = \textbf{6 mL}$

Give 6 mL

Select 10 cc syringe

34. $\dfrac{5000 \text{ U}}{1 \text{ mL}} = \dfrac{4000 \text{ U}}{X \text{ mL}}$

$5000X = 4000$

$\dfrac{5000X}{5000} = \dfrac{4\cancel{000}}{5\cancel{000}}$

$X = \dfrac{4}{5} = \textbf{0.8 mL}$

Give 0.8 mL

Select 1 mL TB or 3 cc syringe

35. $\dfrac{20 \text{ mg}}{1 \text{ mL}} = \dfrac{30 \text{ mg}}{X \text{ mL}}$

$20X = 30$

$\dfrac{20X}{20} = \dfrac{30}{2\cancel{0}}$

$X = \textbf{1.5 mL}$

Give 1.5 mL

Select 3 cc syringe

36. Calcium gluconate 10% = 10 g per 100 mL of solution.

$\dfrac{10 \text{ g}}{100 \text{ mL}} = \dfrac{0.5 \text{ g}}{X \text{ mL}}$

$10X = 50$

$\dfrac{10X}{10} = \dfrac{50}{10}$

$X = \textbf{5 mL}$

Give 5 mL

Select 5 cc syringe

37. $\dfrac{300,000 \text{ U}}{1 \text{ mL}} = \dfrac{400,000 \text{ U}}{X \text{ mL}}$

$300,000X = 400,000$

$\dfrac{300,000X}{300,000} = \dfrac{4\cancel{00,000}}{3\cancel{00,000}}$

$X = \dfrac{4}{3} = 1\dfrac{1}{3}$

$X = \textbf{1.3 mL}$

Give 1.3 mL

Select 3 cc syringe

38. $\dfrac{10 \text{ mg}}{4 \text{ mL}} = \dfrac{2.5 \text{ mg}}{X \text{ mL}}$

$10X = 10$

$\dfrac{10X}{10} = \dfrac{10}{10}$

$X = \textbf{1 mL}$

Give 1 mL

Select 3 cc syringe

39. $\dfrac{5000 \text{ U}}{1 \text{ mL}} = \dfrac{3500 \text{ U}}{X \text{ mL}}$

$5000X = 3500$

$\dfrac{5000X}{5000} = \dfrac{35\cancel{00}}{50\cancel{00}}$

$X = \dfrac{35}{50} = \dfrac{7}{10} = \textbf{0.7 mL}$

Give 0.7 mL

Select 1 mL TB or 3 cc syringe

40. Neostigmine 1:2000 = 1 g in 2000 mL.

$\dfrac{1 \text{ g}}{2000 \text{ mL}} = \dfrac{1000 \text{ mg}}{2000 \text{ mL}} = \dfrac{1 \text{ mg}}{2 \text{ mL}}$

$\dfrac{1 \text{ mg}}{2 \text{ mL}} = \dfrac{0.5 \text{ mg}}{X \text{ mL}}$

$X = \textbf{1 mL}$

Give 1 mL

Select 3 cc syringe

41. $\dfrac{2 \text{ mEq}}{1 \text{ mL}} = \dfrac{60 \text{ mEq}}{X \text{ mL}}$

$2X = 60$

$\dfrac{2X}{2} = \dfrac{60}{2}$

$X = \textbf{30 mL}$

Give 30 mL

Select 2 20 cc syringes

42. **Give 16 U**

Select 30 U or 50 U Lo-Dose syringes

43. **Give 70 units**

Select 100 U Standard U-100 insulin syringe

44. **Give 25 units**

Select 50 U Lo-Dose U-100 insulin syringe

45. $\dfrac{50 \text{ mg}}{1 \text{ mL}} = \dfrac{35 \text{ mg}}{X \text{ mL}}$

$50X = 35$

$\dfrac{50X}{50} = \dfrac{35}{50}$ (7 over, 10 under)

$X = \textbf{0.7 mL}$

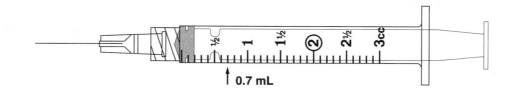

↑ **0.7 mL**

46. $\dfrac{225 \text{ mg}}{1 \text{ mL}} = \dfrac{500 \text{ mg}}{X \text{ mL}}$

$225X = 500$

$\dfrac{225X}{225} = \dfrac{500}{225}$

$X = \textbf{2.2 mL}$

$$\begin{array}{r} 2.22 \\ 225\overline{)500.00} \\ -450 \\ \hline 500 \\ -450 \\ \hline 500 \\ -450 \\ \hline 50 \end{array}$$

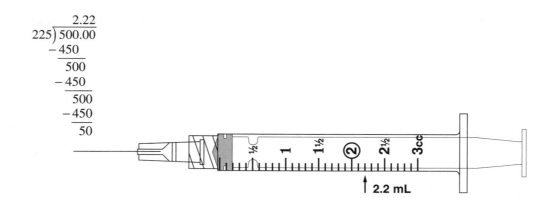

↑ **2.2 mL**

47. $\dfrac{80 \text{ mg}}{2 \text{ mL}} = \dfrac{65 \text{ mg}}{X \text{ mL}}$

$80X = 130$

$\dfrac{80X}{80} = \dfrac{130}{80}$

$X = \textbf{1.6 mL}$

$$\begin{array}{r} 1.62 \\ 8\overline{)13.00} \\ -8 \\ \hline 50 \\ -48 \\ \hline 20 \\ -16 \\ \hline 4 \end{array}$$

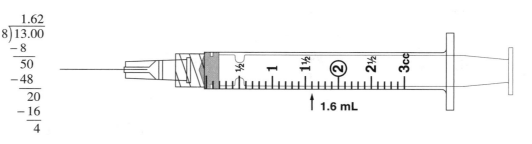

↑ **1.6 mL**

48. If 4.0 mL of diluent is added,

$\dfrac{1 \text{ g}}{2.5 \text{ mL}} = \dfrac{2 \text{ mg}}{X \text{ mL}}$

$X = \textbf{5 mL}$

Give 5 mL

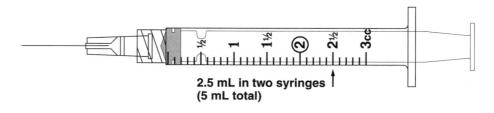

2.5 mL in two syringes ↑
(5 mL total)

49. $\dfrac{1 \text{ mg}}{1 \text{ mL}} = \dfrac{0.5 \text{ mg}}{X \text{ mL}}$

$X = \textbf{0.5 mL}$

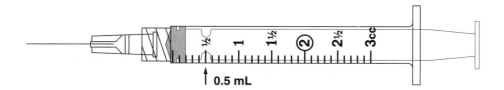

↑ **0.5 mL**

50. $\dfrac{300,000 \text{ U}}{1 \text{ mL}} = \dfrac{400,000 \text{ U}}{X \text{ mL}}$

$300,000X = 400,000$

$\dfrac{300,000X}{300,000} = \dfrac{400,000}{300,000}$

$X = \dfrac{4}{3} = \textbf{1.3 mL}$

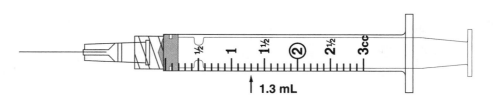

↑ **1.3 mL**

51. **Give 22 units in Lo-Dose 50 U syringe.**

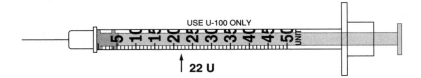

↑ **22 U**

52. $\dfrac{10 \text{ mg}}{1 \text{ mL}} = \dfrac{15 \text{ mg}}{X \text{ mL}}$

$10X = 15$

$\dfrac{10X}{10} = \dfrac{15}{10}$

$X = \textbf{1.5 mL}$

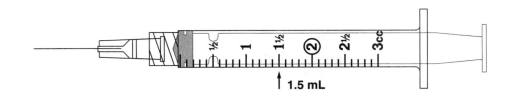

↑ **1.5 mL**

53. $\dfrac{10{,}000 \text{ U}}{1 \text{ mL}} = \dfrac{8000 \text{ U}}{X \text{ mL}}$

$10{,}000X = 8000$

$\dfrac{10{,}000X}{10{,}000} = \dfrac{8000}{10{,}000}$

$X = \textbf{0.8 mL}$

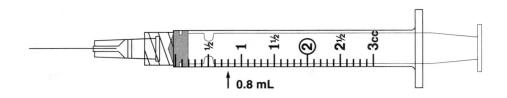

↑ **0.8 mL**

54. $\dfrac{280 \text{ mg}}{1 \text{ mL}} = \dfrac{300 \text{ mg}}{X \text{ mL}}$

$280X = 300$

$\dfrac{280X}{280} = \dfrac{300}{280}$

$X = \textbf{1.1 mL}$

$$\begin{array}{r} 1.07 \\ 28\overline{)30.00} \\ -28 \\ \hline 200 \\ -196 \\ \hline 4 \end{array}$$

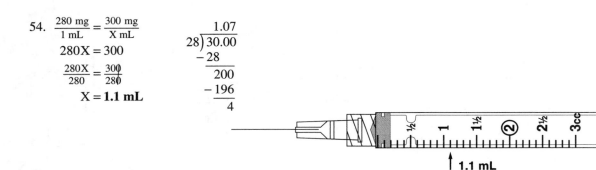

↑ **1.1 mL**

55. $0.5 \text{ g} = 0.5 \times 1000 = 500 \text{ mg}$

$\dfrac{270 \text{ mg}}{1 \text{ mL}} = \dfrac{500 \text{ mg}}{X \text{ mL}}$

$270X = 500$

$\dfrac{270X}{270} = \dfrac{500}{270}$

$X = \textbf{1.9 mL}$

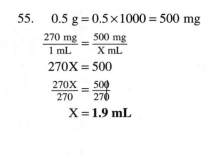

$$\begin{array}{r} 1.85 \\ 27\overline{)50.00} \\ -27 \\ \hline 230 \\ -216 \\ \hline 140 \\ -130 \\ \hline 10 \end{array}$$

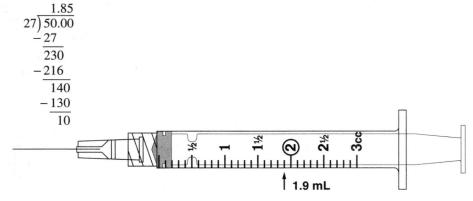

↑ **1.9 mL**

56. $\dfrac{125 \text{ mg}}{1 \text{ mL}} = \dfrac{200 \text{ mg}}{X \text{ mL}}$

$125X = 200$

$\dfrac{125X}{125} = \dfrac{200}{125} = \dfrac{8}{5} = 1\dfrac{3}{5} = 1.6$

$X = \textbf{1.6 mL}$

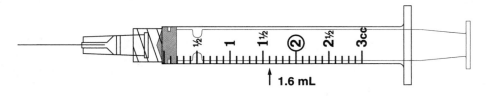

↑ **1.6 mL**

57. $\dfrac{250 \text{ mg}}{1 \text{ mL}} = \dfrac{500 \text{ mg}}{X \text{ mL}}$

$250X = 500$

$\dfrac{250X}{250} = \dfrac{500}{250}$

$X = \textbf{2 mL}$

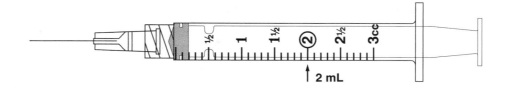

↑ **2 mL**

58. Convert gr $\dfrac{1}{300}$ to mg.

$\dfrac{\text{gr i}}{60 \text{ mg}} = \dfrac{\text{gr } \frac{1}{300}}{X \text{ mg}}$

$X = \dfrac{1}{30\cancel{0}} \times 6\cancel{0}$

$X = \dfrac{1}{5} = 0.2 \text{ mg}$

$\dfrac{0.4 \text{ mg}}{1 \text{ mL}} = \dfrac{0.2 \text{ mg}}{X \text{ mL}}$

$0.4X = 0.2$

$\dfrac{0.4X}{0.4} = \dfrac{0.2}{0.4} = \dfrac{2}{4} = \dfrac{1}{2}$

$X = \textbf{0.5 mL}$

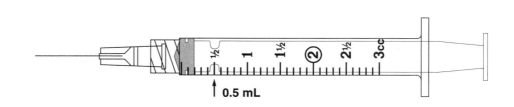

↑ **0.5 mL**

59. $\dfrac{50 \text{ mg}}{1 \text{ mL}} = \dfrac{60 \text{ mg}}{X \text{ mL}}$

$50X = 60$

$\dfrac{50X}{50} = \dfrac{6\cancel{0}}{5\cancel{0}}$

$X = \dfrac{6}{5} = 1\dfrac{1}{5} = \textbf{1.2 mL}$

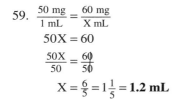 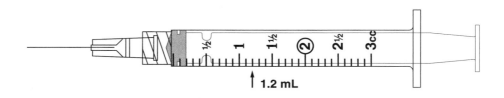

↑ **1.2 mL**

60. $\dfrac{1 \text{ mg}}{1 \text{ mL}} = \dfrac{0.25 \text{ mg}}{X \text{ mL}}$

$X = \textbf{0.25 mL}$

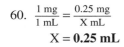 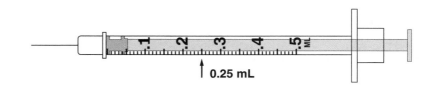

↑ **0.25 mL**

61. **32 U regular insulin**
    54 U NPH insulin

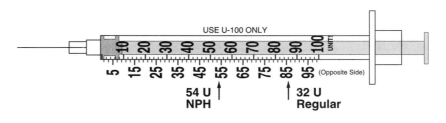

54 U ↑   ↑ **32 U**
NPH   **Regular**

62. **46 U**

 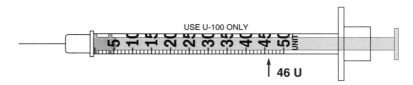

↑ **46 U**

Review Set 27 (page 178)

1. $\dfrac{D}{H} \times Q = X$

    $\dfrac{1.25 \text{ mg}}{0.625 \text{ mg}} \times 1 \text{ tablet} = \textbf{2 tablets}$

2. $\dfrac{D}{H} \times Q = X$

    $\dfrac{\overset{1}{\cancel{150}} \text{ mg}}{\underset{2}{\cancel{300}} \text{ mg}} \times 5 \text{ mL} = \textbf{2.5 mL}$

3. $\dfrac{80 \text{ mg}}{100 \text{ mg}} \times 1 \text{ mL} = \textbf{0.8 mL}$

4. $\dfrac{\overset{7}{\cancel{35}} \text{ mg}}{\underset{10}{\cancel{50}} \text{ mg}} \times 1 \text{ mL} = \textbf{0.7 mL}$

5. $\dfrac{\overset{3}{\cancel{12}} \text{ mEq}}{\underset{2}{\cancel{8}} \text{ mEq}} \times 5 \text{ mL} = \dfrac{15}{2} = \textbf{7.5 mL}$

6. $\dfrac{2.4 \text{ mg}}{4 \text{ mg}} \times 1 \text{ mL} = \textbf{0.6 mL}$

7. $\dfrac{D}{H} \times Q = X$

    $\dfrac{7.5 \text{ mg}}{5 \text{ mg}} \times 1 \text{ tab} = 1.5 = \textbf{1}\frac{1}{2}\textbf{ tablets}$

8. $\dfrac{30 \text{ mg}}{\underset{30}{\cancel{50}} \text{ mg}} \times \overset{1}{\cancel{5}} \text{ mL} = \textbf{3 mL}$

9. $\dfrac{\overset{2}{\cancel{160}} \text{ mg}}{\underset{1}{\cancel{80}} \text{ mg}} \times 15 \text{ mL} = \textbf{30 mL}$

10. $\dfrac{\overset{4}{\cancel{20}} \text{ mg}}{\underset{5}{\cancel{25}} \text{ mg}} \times 2 \text{ mL} = \dfrac{8}{5} = 1\frac{3}{5} = \textbf{1.6 mL}$

11. $\dfrac{15 \text{ mg}}{\underset{5}{\cancel{25}} \text{ mg}} \times \overset{1}{\cancel{5}} \text{ mL} = \textbf{3 mL}$

12. $\dfrac{2 \text{ mg}}{4 \text{ mg}} \times 1 \text{ mL} = \textbf{0.5 mL}$

13. $\text{gr ss} = \frac{1}{2} \times 60 = \textbf{30 mg}$

    $\dfrac{30 \text{ mg}}{15 \text{ mg}} \times 1 \text{ tab} = \textbf{2 tablets}$

14. $\dfrac{125 \text{ mg}}{250 \text{ mg}} \times 1 \text{ tab} = \frac{1}{2} \text{ tablet}$

    Give $\frac{1}{2}$ of the 250 mg tablet.

15. $\dfrac{\overset{12}{\cancel{60}} \text{ mg}}{\underset{5}{\cancel{25}} \text{ mg}} \times 1 \text{ mL} = \dfrac{12}{5} = 2\frac{2}{5} = \textbf{2.4 mL}$

16. $0.15 \text{ mg} = 0.15 \times 1000 = 150 \text{ mcg}$

    $\dfrac{150 \text{ mcg}}{75 \text{ mcg}} \times 1 \text{ tab} = \textbf{2 tablets}$

17. $\dfrac{\cancel{160} \text{ mg}}{\underset{2}{\cancel{100}} \text{ mg}} \times \overset{1}{\cancel{5}} \text{ mL} = \textbf{8 mL}$

18. $\dfrac{100 \text{ mg}}{80 \text{ mg}} \times 1 \text{ mL} = \dfrac{5}{4} = 1\frac{1}{4} = 1.25$

    $= \textbf{1.3 mL}$ measured in 3 cc syringe.

19. $\dfrac{8 \text{ mg}}{2.5 \text{ mg}} \times 5 \text{ mL} = \dfrac{40}{2.5} = \textbf{16 mL}$

    $\begin{array}{r} 16. \\ 2.5\overline{)40.0} \\ -25 \\ \hline 150 \\ -150 \\ \hline 0 \end{array}$

20. $\dfrac{350 \text{ mg}}{\underset{5}{\cancel{250}} \text{ mg}} \times \overset{1}{\cancel{5}} \text{ mL} = \textbf{7mL}$

Practice Problems—Chapter 9 (page 180)

1. $\dfrac{D}{H} \times Q = X$

    $\dfrac{\overset{1}{\cancel{30}} \text{ g}}{\underset{1.11}{\cancel{3.33}} \text{ g}} \times 5 \text{ mL} = \dfrac{50}{1.11}$

    $X = 45 \text{ mL}$

    $\begin{array}{r} 45.0 \\ 1.11\overline{)50.00.0} \\ -444 \\ \hline 560 \\ -555 \\ \hline 50 \end{array}$

    Give 45 mL

2. $\dfrac{D}{H} \times Q = X$

    $\dfrac{\overset{1}{\cancel{600,000}} \text{ U}}{\underset{1}{\cancel{3,000,000}} \text{ U}} \times 2\cancel{0} \text{ mL} = 2 \text{ mL}$

    Give 2 mL

3. $\dfrac{8\cancel{0} \text{ mg}}{\underset{5}{\cancel{250}} \text{ mg}} \times \overset{1}{\cancel{5}} \text{ mL} = \dfrac{8}{5} = 1\frac{3}{5} = \textbf{1.6 mL}$

    Give 1.6 mL

4. $\dfrac{\overset{1}{\cancel{125} \text{ mg}}}{\underset{2}{\cancel{250} \text{ mg}}} \times 5 \text{ mL} = 2.5 \text{ mL}$ $2.5 \text{ mL} = \dfrac{2.5}{5} = \dfrac{1}{2} \text{ t}$

Give $\dfrac{1}{2}$ teaspoon

5. $\dfrac{\overset{5}{\cancel{25} \text{ mg}}}{\underset{2}{\cancel{10} \text{ mg}}} \times 1 \text{ mL} = 2.5 \text{ mL}$

Give 2.5 mL

6. $\dfrac{40 \text{ mg}}{\underset{2.5}{\cancel{12.5} \text{ mg}}} \times \overset{1}{\cancel{5}} \text{ mL} = 16 \text{ mL}$

$$2.5\overline{)40.0} \quad \begin{array}{r} 16. \\ \hline \end{array}$$
$$\begin{array}{r} -25 \\ \hline 150 \\ -150 \\ \hline 0 \end{array}$$

Give 16 mL

7. $\dfrac{\overset{7}{\cancel{350,000} \text{ U}}}{\underset{10}{\cancel{500,000} \text{ U}}} \times 2 \text{ mL} = 1.4 \text{ mL}$

Give 1.4 mL

8. $\dfrac{3.5 \text{ mg}}{10 \text{ mg}} \times 2 \text{ mL} = 0.7 \text{ mL}$

Give 0.7 mL

9. $\dfrac{\overset{9}{\cancel{90} \text{ mg}}}{\underset{4}{\cancel{80} \text{ mg}}} \times \overset{1}{\cancel{2}} \text{ mL} = \dfrac{9}{4} = 2\dfrac{1}{4} = 2.25 = 2.3 \text{ mL}$

Give 2.3 mL

10. $\dfrac{2,500 \text{ U}}{20,000 \text{ U}} \times 1 \text{ mL} = \dfrac{25}{200} = \dfrac{1}{8} = 0.125 = 0.13 \text{ mL}$

Give 0.13 mL measured in a tuberculin syringe.

11. $\dfrac{8 \text{ mg}}{10 \text{ mg}} \times 2 \text{ mL} = 1.6 \text{ mL}$

Give 1.6 mL

12. $\dfrac{\cancel{60} \text{ mg}}{\underset{4}{\cancel{80} \text{ mg}}} \times \overset{1}{\cancel{2}} \text{ mL} = \dfrac{3}{2} = 1.5 \text{ mL}$

Give 1.5 mL

13. $\dfrac{\overset{1}{\cancel{500} \text{ mg}}}{\underset{2}{\cancel{1000} \text{ mg}}} \times 2.5 \text{ mL} = 1.25 = 1.3 \text{ mL}$

Give 1.3 mL

14. $\dfrac{250,000 \text{ U}}{100,000 \text{ U}} \times 1 \text{ mL} = 2.5 \text{ mL}$

Give 2.5 mL

15. $\dfrac{80 \text{ mg}}{\underset{5}{\cancel{250} \text{ mg}}} \times \overset{1}{\cancel{5}} \text{ mL} = \dfrac{8}{5} = 1\dfrac{3}{5} = 1.6 \text{ mL}$

Give 1.6 mL

16. $\dfrac{\cancel{10} \text{ mEq}}{\cancel{20} \text{ mEq}} \times 15 \text{ mL} = 7.5 \text{ mL}$

Give 7.5 mL

17. $1 \text{ g} = 1000 \text{ mg}$

$\dfrac{\cancel{400} \text{ mg}}{\cancel{1000} \text{ mg}} \times 4 \text{ mL} = \dfrac{160}{100} = 1.6 \text{ mL}$

Give 1.6 mL

18. $0.075 \text{ mg} = 0.075 \times 1000 = 75 \text{ mcg}$

$\dfrac{150 \text{ mcg}}{75 \text{ mcg}} \times 1 \text{ tab} = 2 \text{ tablets}$

Give 2 tablets

19. $\dfrac{400 \text{ mg}}{\underset{5}{\cancel{250} \text{ mg}}} \times \overset{1}{\cancel{5}} \text{ mL} = 8 \text{ mL}$

Give 8 mL

20. $\dfrac{\overset{9}{\cancel{225} \text{ mg}}}{\underset{2}{\cancel{50} \text{ mg}}} \times 1 \text{ mL} = \dfrac{9}{2} = 4\dfrac{1}{2} = 4.5 \text{ mL}$

Give 4.5 mL

21. $\dfrac{\overset{2}{\cancel{160} \text{ mg}}}{\underset{1}{\cancel{80} \text{ mg}}} \times 15 \text{ mL} = 30 \text{ mL}$

Give 30 mL

22. $\dfrac{\overset{7}{\cancel{35} \text{ mg}}}{\underset{5}{\cancel{25} \text{ mg}}} \times 1 \text{ mL} = \dfrac{7}{5} = 1\dfrac{2}{5} = 1.4$

Give 1.4 mL

23. $\dfrac{30 \text{ mEq}}{\underset{2}{\cancel{40} \text{ mEq}}} \times \overset{1}{\cancel{20}} \text{ mL} = 15 \text{ mL}$

Add 15 mL

24. $\dfrac{25 \text{ mg}}{\underset{1.25}{\cancel{6.25} \text{ mg}}} \times \overset{1}{\cancel{5}} \text{ mL} = \dfrac{25}{1.25} = 20 \text{ mL}$

$$1.25\overline{)25.00} \quad \begin{array}{r} 20. \\ \hline \end{array}$$
$$\begin{array}{r} -250 \\ \hline 00 \end{array}$$

Give 20 mL

25. $\dfrac{300 \text{ mg}}{\underset{25}{\cancel{125} \text{ mg}}} \times \overset{1}{\cancel{5}} \text{ mL} = 12 \text{ mL}$

Give 12 mL

Review Set 28 (page 191)

1. $55 \text{ lb} = \frac{55}{2.2} = 25 \text{ kg}$

   per day, $\frac{25 \text{ mg}}{1 \text{ kg}} = \frac{X \text{ mg}}{25 \text{ kg}}$

   $X = 625 \text{ mg}$

   $625 \text{ mg/day divided q.6h} = \frac{625 \text{ mg}}{4}$

   $= 156.25 = \textbf{156 mg}$

2. $\frac{62.5 \text{ mg}}{5 \text{ mL}} = \frac{156 \text{ mg}}{X \text{ mL}}$

   $62.5X = 780$

   $\frac{62.5X}{62.5} = \frac{780}{62.5}$

   $X = \textbf{12.5 mL}$

$$
\begin{array}{r}
12.48 \\
62.5\overline{)780.000} \\
-625 \\
\hline
1550 \\
-1250 \\
\hline
3000 \\
-2500 \\
\hline
5000 \\
-5000 \\
\hline
0
\end{array}
$$

3. $2000 \text{ g} = 2 \text{ kg}$

   per day, $\frac{25 \text{ mg}}{1 \text{ kg}} = \frac{X \text{ mg}}{2 \text{ kg}}$

   $X = 50 \text{ mg}$

   $50 \text{ mg/day divided in 2 doses} = \frac{50 \text{ mg}}{2} = \textbf{25 mg}$

4. $\frac{100 \text{ mg}}{1 \text{ mL}} = \frac{25 \text{ mg}}{X \text{ mL}}$

   $100X = 25$

   $\frac{100X}{100} = \frac{25}{100}$

   $X = \textbf{0.25 mL}$

5. $33 \text{ lb} = \frac{33}{2.2} = 15 \text{ kg}$

   per day: $\frac{100 \text{ mg}}{1 \text{ kg}} = \frac{X \text{ mg}}{15 \text{ kg}}$

   $X = 1500 \text{ mg}$

   $1500 \text{ mg/day divided q.i.d.} = \frac{1500 \text{ mg}}{4} = \textbf{375 mg}$

6. $1 \text{ g} = 1000 \text{ mg}$

   $\frac{1000 \text{ mg}}{4 \text{ mL}} = \frac{375 \text{ mg}}{X \text{ mL}}$

   $\frac{1000X}{1000} = \frac{1500}{1000}$

   $X = \textbf{1.5 mL}$

7. per dose: $\frac{10 \text{ mg}}{1 \text{ kg}} = \frac{X \text{ mg}}{32 \text{ kg}}$

   $X = 320 \text{ mg}$

   $\frac{160 \text{ mg}}{1 \text{ mL}} = \frac{320 \text{ mg}}{X \text{ mL}}$

   $160X = 320$

   $\frac{160X}{160} = \frac{320}{160}$

   $X = 2 \text{ mL}$

   Give 2 mL

8. $4000 \text{ g} = 4 \text{ kg}$

   per day: $\frac{4 \text{ mg}}{1 \text{ kg}} = \frac{X \text{ mg}}{4 \text{ kg}}$

   $X = 16 \text{ mg}$

   $16 \text{ mg/day divided every 12 hours} = \frac{16 \text{ mg}}{2} = \textbf{8 mg}$

9. $\frac{40 \text{ mg}}{1 \text{ mL}} = \frac{8 \text{ mg}}{X \text{ mL}}$

   $40X = 8$

   $\frac{40X}{40} = \frac{8}{40}$

   $X = \frac{1}{5} = \textbf{0.2 mL}$

10. $44 \text{ lb} = \frac{44}{2.2} = 20 \text{ kg}$

    per day: $\frac{25 \text{ mg}}{1 \text{ kg}} = \frac{X \text{ mg}}{20 \text{ kg}}$

    $X = 500 \text{ mg}$

    $500 \text{ mg/day divided in four doses} = \frac{500 \text{ mg}}{4} = \textbf{125 mg}$

    $\frac{250 \text{ mg}}{5 \text{ mL}} = \frac{125 \text{ mg}}{X \text{ mL}}$

    $250X = 625$

    $\frac{250X}{250} = \frac{625}{250}$

    $X = 2.5 \text{ mL}$

$$
\begin{array}{r}
2.5 \\
250\overline{)625.0} \\
-500 \\
\hline
1250 \\
-1250 \\
\hline
0
\end{array}
$$

    Give 2.5 mL

11. **20 to 40 mg/kg/day** in divided doses every 8 hours

12. **3 doses daily (q.8h = 3 doses in 24 hr)**

13. $15 \text{ lb} = \frac{15}{2.2} = 6.8 \text{ kg}$

$$\begin{array}{r} 6.8 \\ 2.2\overline{)15.00} \\ -132 \\ \hline 180 \\ -176 \\ \hline 4 \end{array}$$

Minimum per day: $\frac{20 \text{ mg}}{1 \text{ kg}} = \frac{X \text{ mg}}{6.8 \text{ kg}}$

$X = 136 \text{ mg}$

136 mg/day divided in 3 doses = 45.33 mg/dose

Maximum per day: $\frac{40 \text{ mg}}{1 \text{ kg}} = \frac{X \text{ mg}}{6.8 \text{ kg}}$

$X = 272 \text{ mg}$

272 mg/day divided in 3 doses = 90.66 mg/dose.

Safe range is 45.33 mg to 90.66 mg/dose.

The ordered amount, 75 mg/dose, is within the recommended range. Yes, it is safe.

14. $\frac{50 \text{ mg}}{1 \text{ mL}} = \frac{75 \text{ mg}}{X \text{ mL}}$

$50X = 75$

$\frac{50X}{50} = \frac{75}{50}$

$X = \frac{3}{2} = \textbf{1.5 mL/dose}$

15. 1.5 mL q.8h × 10 days

$\frac{1.5 \text{ mL}}{\text{dose}} \times \frac{3 \text{ doses}}{\text{day}} \times 10 \text{ days} = 45 \text{ mL}$

No, one 15 mL bottle is not enough to administer the full 10 day order. Three 15 mL bottles would be needed.

16. **5 mg/kg/day or 60 mg/day in 2 equally divided dosages.**

17. $9 \text{ lb} = \frac{9}{2.2} = 4 \text{ kg}$

per day, $\frac{15 \text{ mg}}{1 \text{ kg}} = \frac{X \text{ mg}}{4 \text{ kg}}$

$X = 60 \text{ mg}$

60 mg/day divided b.i.d = $\frac{60 \text{ mg}}{2} = 30$ mg/dose.

Yes, the order of 30 mg b.i.d is safe.

18. $\frac{75 \text{ mg}}{2 \text{ mL}} = \frac{30 \text{ mg}}{X \text{ mL}}$

$75X = 60$

$\frac{75X}{75} = \frac{60}{75}$

$X = \frac{4}{5} = \textbf{0.8 mL}$

19. per day, minimum: $\frac{100 \text{ mg}}{1 \text{ kg}} = \frac{X \text{ mg}}{8 \text{ kg}}$

$X = \textbf{800 mg}$

20. per day, maximum: $\frac{200 \text{ mg}}{1 \text{ kg}} = \frac{X \text{ mg}}{8 \text{ kg}}$

$X = \textbf{1600 mg}$

21. Safe range if ordered q.6h

minimum : $\frac{800 \text{ mg}}{4} = \textbf{200 mg/dose}$

maximum : $\frac{1600 \text{ mg}}{4} = \textbf{400 mg/dose}$

22. **Yes, it is safe.**

23. Safe range of TMP/day:

minimum : $\frac{6 \text{ mg}}{1 \text{ kg}} = \frac{X \text{ mg}}{15 \text{ kg}}$

$X = 90 \text{ mg}$

maximum : $\frac{12 \text{ mg}}{1 \text{ kg}} = \frac{X \text{ mg}}{15 \text{ mg}}$

$X = 180 \text{ mg}$

The 15 kg child could receive 90–180 mg of the TMP component of Septra daily.

24. $\frac{16 \text{ mg}}{1 \text{ mL}} = \frac{X \text{ mg}}{5.6 \text{ mL}} =$

$X = 89.6$ or 90 mg of TMP q.12h

Yes, it is safe.

Review Set 29 (page 195)

1. **0.56 m^2**

2. 1 g = 1000 mg

$\frac{\text{Child BSA}}{1.7} \times \text{Adult dose} = \frac{0.56}{1.7} \times 1000 \text{ mg}$

$= \textbf{330 mg}$

3. BSA = 0.27 m^2

   $\dfrac{0.27}{1.7} \times 250$ mg $= 39.7 =$ **40 mg**

4. **1 m^2**

5. $\dfrac{250 \text{ mg}}{\text{m}^2} \times 1.0$ m$^2 =$ **250 mg**

6. 30 inches, 25 pounds = 0.5 m^2 BSA

   $\dfrac{250 \text{ mg}}{\text{m}^2} \times 0.5$ m$^2 = 125$ mg

   $\dfrac{D}{H} \times Q = \dfrac{125 \text{ mg}}{50 \text{ mg}} \times 1$ mL $=$ **2.5 mL**

   or, $\dfrac{50 \text{ mg}}{1 \text{ mL}} = \dfrac{125 \text{ mg}}{X \text{ mL}}$

   $\quad 50X = 125$

   $\quad \dfrac{50X}{50} = \dfrac{125}{50}$

   $\quad\quad X = \dfrac{125}{50} = \dfrac{5}{2}$

   $\quad\quad X = 2.5$ mL

7. 45 inches, 55 pounds = 0.9 m^2 BSA

   $\dfrac{0.3 \text{ mg}}{\text{m}^2} \times 0.9$ m$^2 = 2.97$ mg (round to 3 mg)

   $\dfrac{D}{H} \times Q = \dfrac{3 \text{ mg}}{5 \text{ mg}} \times 2$ mL $= \dfrac{6}{5} =$ **1.2 mL**

   or, $\dfrac{5 \text{ mg}}{2 \text{ mL}} = \dfrac{3 \text{ mg}}{X \text{ mL}}$

   $\quad 5X = 6$

   $\quad \dfrac{5X}{5} = \dfrac{6}{5}$

   $\quad\quad X = \dfrac{6}{5}$

   $\quad\quad X = 1.2$ mL

8. BSA = 0.8 m^2

   $\dfrac{0.8 \text{ m}^2}{1.7 \text{ m}^2} \times 500$ mg $=$ **235 mg**

Practice Problems—Chapter 10 (page 198)

1. 20 lb $= \dfrac{20}{2.2} = 9$ kg

   $\dfrac{2 \text{ mg}}{1 \text{ kg}} = \dfrac{X \text{ mg}}{9 \text{ kg}}$

   $\quad X = 18$ mg

   $\dfrac{20 \text{ mg}}{2 \text{ mL}} = \dfrac{18 \text{ mg}}{X \text{ mL}}$

   $\quad 20X = 36$

   $\quad \dfrac{20X}{20} = \dfrac{36}{20} = \dfrac{18}{10}$

   $\quad\quad X =$ **1.8 mL**

2. 66 lb $= \dfrac{66}{2.2} = 30$ kg

   $\dfrac{3 \text{ mg}}{1 \text{ kg}} = \dfrac{X \text{ mg}}{30 \text{ kg}}$

   $\quad X = 90$ mg

   Order is for 105 mg.

   Recommended dose is 90 mg.

   Order is for more than recommended dosage.

   Consult with physician or your supervisor before administering.

3. Child's BSA = 0.52 m^2

   $\dfrac{0.52 \text{ m}^2}{1.7 \text{ m}^2} \times 100$ mg $= 31$ mg

   $\dfrac{50 \text{ mg}}{1 \text{ mL}} = \dfrac{31 \text{ mg}}{X \text{ mL}}$

   $\quad 50X = 31$

   $\quad \dfrac{50X}{50} = \dfrac{31}{50} = \dfrac{62}{100}$

   $\quad\quad X =$ **0.62 mL**

4. Child's BSA = 0.42 m^2

   $\dfrac{0.42 \text{ m}^2}{1.7 \text{ m}^2} \times 500$ mg $=$ **125 mg**

5. $\dfrac{250 \text{ mg}}{1 \text{ mL}} = \dfrac{125 \text{ mg}}{X \text{ mL}}$

   $\quad 250X = 125$

   $\quad \dfrac{250X}{250} = \dfrac{125}{250}$

   $\quad\quad X =$ **0.5 mL**

6. Child's BSA = 0.6 m^2

   $\dfrac{0.6 \text{ m}^2}{1.7 \text{ m}^2} \times 500$ mg $=$ **175 mg**

7. $\dfrac{250 \text{ mg}}{1 \text{ mL}} = \dfrac{175 \text{ mg}}{X \text{ mL}}$

   $\quad 250X = 175$

   $\quad \dfrac{250X}{250} = \dfrac{175}{250} = \dfrac{7}{10}$

   $\quad\quad X =$ **0.7 mL**

8. BSA = 0.8 m^2

   $\dfrac{0.8 \text{ m}^2}{1.7 \text{ m}^2} \times 500$ mg $=$ **235 mg**

9. $\dfrac{250 \text{ mg}}{1 \text{ mL}} = \dfrac{235 \text{ mg}}{X \text{ mL}}$

   $250X = 235$

   $\dfrac{250X}{250} = \dfrac{235}{250}$

   $X = \textbf{0.94 mL}$

10. $55 \text{ lb} = \dfrac{55}{2.2} = 25 \text{ kg}$

    $\dfrac{0.2 \text{ g}}{1 \text{ kg}} = \dfrac{X \text{ g}}{25 \text{ kg}}$

    $X = 5 \text{ g}$

    $\dfrac{6 \text{ g}}{100 \text{ mL}} = \dfrac{5 \text{ g}}{X \text{ mL}}$

    $6X = 500$

    $\dfrac{6X}{6} = \dfrac{500}{6}$

    $X = \textbf{83 mL}$

11. $26 \text{ lb} = \dfrac{26}{2.2} = 12 \text{ kg}$

    per day, $\dfrac{50 \text{ mg}}{1 \text{ kg}} = \dfrac{X \text{ mg}}{12 \text{ kg}}$

    $X = 600 \text{ mg}$

    600 mg/day divided q.6h = $\dfrac{600 \text{ mg}}{4} = 150 \text{ mg/dose}$

    $\dfrac{D}{H} \times Q = \dfrac{150 \text{ mg}}{125 \text{ mg}} \times 5 \text{ mL} = \textbf{6 mL}$

    $\dfrac{125 \text{ mg}}{5 \text{ mL}} = \dfrac{150 \text{ mg}}{X \text{ mL}}$

    $125X = 750$

    $\dfrac{125X}{125} = \dfrac{750}{125} = \dfrac{30}{5} = 6$

    $X = 6 \text{ mL}$

12. $BSA = 1.3 \text{ m}^2$

    $\dfrac{20 \text{ mg}}{\text{m}^2} \times 1.3 \text{ m}^2 = 26 \text{ mg}$

    $\dfrac{2 \text{ mg}}{1 \text{ mL}} = \dfrac{26 \text{ mg}}{X \text{ mL}}$

    $2X = 26$

    $\dfrac{2X}{2} = \dfrac{26}{2}$

    $X = \textbf{13 mL}$ or

    $\dfrac{D}{H} \times Q = \dfrac{26 \text{ mg}}{2 \text{ mg}} \times 1 \text{ mL} = \textbf{13 mL}$

13. 45 inches, 55 pounds = 0.9 m² BSA

    $\dfrac{2 \text{ mg}}{\text{m}^2} \times 0.9 \text{ m}^2 = 1.8 \text{ mg}$

    $\dfrac{D}{H} \times Q = \dfrac{1.8 \text{ mg}}{1 \text{ mg}} \times 1 \text{ mL} = \textbf{1.8 mL}$

    or, $\dfrac{1 \text{ mg}}{1 \text{ mL}} = \dfrac{1.8 \text{ mg}}{X \text{ mL}}$

    $X = 1.8 \text{ mL}$

14. $11 \text{ lb} = \dfrac{11}{2.2} = \textbf{5 kg}$

15. **75 mg** daily

    per day, $\dfrac{15 \text{ mg}}{1 \text{ kg}} = \dfrac{X \text{ mg}}{5 \text{ kg}}$

    $X = 75 \text{ mg}$

16. 75 mg divided q.12h = $\dfrac{75 \text{ mg}}{2} = \textbf{37.5 mg}$

17. **Yes**

18. $\dfrac{75 \text{ mg}}{2 \text{ mL}} = \dfrac{37.5 \text{ mg}}{X \text{ mL}}$

    $75X = 75$

    $\dfrac{75X}{75} = \dfrac{75}{75}$

    $X = 1 \text{ mL}$ or

    $\dfrac{37.5 \text{ mg}}{75 \text{ mg}} \times 2 \text{ mL} = \dfrac{75 \text{ mg}}{75 \text{ mg}} = \textbf{1 mL}$

19. **Yes,** it is safe.

    $22 \text{ lb} = \dfrac{22}{2.2} = 10 \text{ kg}$

    per day, $10 \text{ kg} \times \dfrac{50 \text{ mg}}{\text{kg}} = 500 \text{ mg}$

    500 mg per day q.6h = $\dfrac{500 \text{ mg}}{4} = 125 \text{ mg per dose}$

20. $44 \text{ lb} = \dfrac{44}{2.2} = 20 \text{ kg}$

    Minimum amount:

    per day, $\dfrac{25 \text{ mg}}{1 \text{ kg}} = \dfrac{X \text{ mg}}{20 \text{ kg}}$

    $X = 500 \text{ mg}$

    500 mg/day divided q.6h = $\dfrac{500 \text{ mg}}{4} = 125 \text{ mg/dose}$

    Maximum amount:

    per day, $\dfrac{50 \text{ mg}}{1 \text{ kg}} = \dfrac{X \text{ mg}}{20 \text{ kg}}$

    $X = 1000 \text{ mg}$

    1000 mg/day divided q.6h = $\dfrac{1000 \text{ mg}}{4} = 250 \text{ mg/dose}$

    Ordered amount of 300 mg q.6h is not safe.

    Contact the physician.

21. $\dfrac{10 \text{ mg}}{1 \text{ kg}} = \dfrac{X \text{ mg}}{12 \text{ kg}}$

    $X = \textbf{120 mg}$

22. $\dfrac{80 \text{ mg}}{2.5 \text{ mL}} = \dfrac{120 \text{ mg}}{X \text{ mL}}$

    $80X = 300$

    $\dfrac{80X}{80} = \dfrac{300}{80}$

    $X = \textbf{3.75 mL}$

23. Minimum amount per day:

    $\dfrac{10 \text{ mcg}}{1 \text{ kg}} = \dfrac{X \text{ mcg}}{4 \text{ kg}}$

    $X = 40 \text{ mcg}$

    Maximum amount per day:

    $\dfrac{12 \text{ mcg}}{1 \text{ kg}} = \dfrac{X \text{ mcg}}{4 \text{ kg}}$

    $X = 48 \text{ mcg}$

    Ordered amount:

    $0.048 \text{ mcg} = 0.048 \times 1000 = 48 \text{ mcg}$

    Yes, it is safe.

24. Minimum amount:

    $\dfrac{0.08 \text{ mg}}{1 \text{ kg}} = \dfrac{X \text{ mg}}{14 \text{ kg}}$

    $X = 1.12 \text{ mg}$

    Maximum amount:

    $\dfrac{0.2 \text{ mg}}{1 \text{ kg}} = \dfrac{X \text{ mg}}{14 \text{ kg}}$

    $X = 2.8 \text{ mg}$

    Ordered amount of 2 mg is within safe range.

25. per dose, $\dfrac{0.001 \text{ mg}}{1 \text{ kg}} = \dfrac{X \text{ mg}}{40 \text{ kg}}$

    $X = \textbf{0.04 mg/dose}$

26. $\dfrac{0.04 \text{ mg}}{0.05 \text{ mg}} \times 1 \text{ mL} = \textbf{0.8 mL}$ or

    $\dfrac{0.05 \text{ mg}}{1 \text{ mL}} = \dfrac{0.04 \text{ mg}}{X \text{ mL}}$

    $0.05X = 0.04$

    $\dfrac{0.05X}{0.05} = \dfrac{0.04}{0.05}$

    $X = \dfrac{4}{5} = 0.8 \text{ mL}$

27. per day, $\dfrac{7.5 \text{ mg}}{1 \text{ kg}} = \dfrac{X \text{ mg}}{15 \text{ kg}}$

    $X = \textbf{112.5 mg/day}$

28. 112.5 mg/day divided q.8h = $\dfrac{112.5 \text{ mg}}{3}$

    $= 37.5 \text{ mg/dose}$

29. 1–2 mg/kg/day for 22 kg child:

    Minimum per day:

    $\dfrac{1 \text{ mg}}{1 \text{ kg}} = \dfrac{X \text{ mg}}{22 \text{ kg}}$

    $X = 22 \text{ mg}$

    Maximum per day:

    $\dfrac{2 \text{ mg}}{1 \text{ kg}} = \dfrac{X \text{ mg}}{22 \text{ kg}}$

    $X = 44 \text{ mg}$

    Safe range is 22–44 mg/day up to 1–2 mg/kg/dose, or 22 mg–44 mg/dose

30. 6 kg and 60 cm = **0.33 m^2**

31. $\dfrac{180 \text{ mg}}{\text{m}^2} \times 0.33 \text{ m}^2 = \textbf{59.4 mg q6h}$

32. Minimum per day:

    $\dfrac{6 \text{ mg}}{1 \text{ kg}} = \dfrac{X \text{ mg}}{25 \text{ kg}}$

    $X = \textbf{150 mg}$

    Maximum per day:

    $\dfrac{12 \text{ mg}}{1 \text{ kg}} = \dfrac{X \text{ mg}}{25 \text{ kg}}$

    $X = \textbf{300 mg}$

33. Minimum per dose:

    150 mg/day divided q.12h = $\dfrac{150 \text{ mg}}{2} = \textbf{75 mg}$

    Maximum/dose:

    300 mg/day divided q.12h = $\dfrac{300 \text{ mg}}{2} = \textbf{150 mg}$

34. $\dfrac{16 \text{ mg}}{1 \text{ mL}} = \dfrac{X \text{ mg}}{9.3 \text{ mL}}$

    $X = 148.8 \text{ mg q.12h}$

    Order is within the recommended range.

    Yes, it is safe.

Review Set 30 (page 205)

1. **normal saline; C**

2. **dextrose 5%, water; E**

3. **dextrose 5%, normal saline (0.9% sodium chloride); G**

4. **dextrose 5%, 0.45% sodium chloride; D**

5. **dextrose 5%, 0.225% sodium chloride; A**

6. **dextrose 5%, Ringer's Lactate; H**

7. **dextrose 5%, 0.45% sodium chloride, potassium chloride 20 mEq per liter; B**

8. **dextrose 5%, normal saline (0.9% sodium chloride), potassium chloride 20 mEq per liter; F**

Review Set 31 (page 209)

1.   5% = 5 g dextrose per 100 mL

$$\frac{5 \text{ g}}{100 \text{ mL}} = \frac{X \text{ g}}{1000 \text{ mL}}$$

$$100X = 5000$$

$$\frac{100X}{100} = \frac{5000}{100}$$

X = 5 g dextrose

0.9% = 0.9 NaCl per 100 mL

$$\frac{0.9 \text{ g}}{100 \text{ mL}} = \frac{X \text{ g}}{1000 \text{ mL}}$$

$$100X = 900$$

$$\frac{100X}{100} = \frac{900}{100}$$

X = 9 g NaCl

2.   5% = 5 g dextrose per 100 mL

$$\frac{5 \text{ g}}{100 \text{ mL}} = \frac{X \text{ g}}{500 \text{ mL}}$$

$$\frac{100X}{100} = \frac{2500}{100}$$

$$100X = 2500$$

X = 25 g dextrose

$\frac{1}{2}$ NS = 0.45% NaCl = 0.45 g NaCl per 100 mL

$$\frac{0.45 \text{ g}}{100 \text{ mL}} = \frac{X \text{ g}}{500 \text{ mL}}$$

$$100X = 225$$

$$\frac{100X}{100} = \frac{225}{100}$$

X = 2.25 g NaCl

3.   10% = 10 g dextrose per 100 mL

$$\frac{10 \text{ g}}{100 \text{ mL}} = \frac{X \text{ g}}{250 \text{ mL}}$$

$$100X = 2500$$

$$\frac{100X}{100} = \frac{2500}{100}$$

X = 25 g dextrose

4.   0.9% = 0.9 g NaCl per 100 mL

$$\frac{0.9 \text{ g}}{100 \text{ mL}} = \frac{X \text{ g}}{750 \text{ mL}}$$

$$100X = 675$$

$$\frac{100X}{100} = \frac{675}{100}$$

X = 6.75 g NaCl

Review Set 32 (page 215)

1.   1 L = 1000 mL

$$\frac{1000 \text{ mL}}{10 \text{ h}} = \textbf{100 mL/h}$$

2. $\frac{1800 \text{ mL}}{15 \text{ hr}} = \textbf{120 mL/h}$

3. $\frac{2000 \text{ mL}}{24 \text{ h}} = 83.33 = \textbf{83 mL/h}$

4. $\frac{100 \text{ mL}}{30 \text{ min}} = \frac{X \text{ mL}}{60 \text{ min}}$

$$30X = 6000$$

$$\frac{30X}{30} = \frac{6000}{30}$$

$$X = \frac{6000}{30} = \textbf{200 mL/h}$$

5. $\frac{30 \text{ mL}}{15 \text{ min}} = \frac{X \text{ mL}}{60 \text{ min}}$

$$15X = 1800$$

$$X = \frac{1800}{15} = \textbf{120 mL/h}$$

6.   2.5 L = 2500 mL

$$\frac{2500 \text{ mL}}{20 \text{ h}} = \textbf{125 mL/h}$$

Review Set 33 (page 216)

1. **15 gtt/mL**

2. **20 gtt/mL**

3. **60 gtt/mL**

4. **60 gtt/mL**

5. **10 gtt/mL**

Review Set 34 (page 218)

1. $\frac{\text{Total Volume}}{\text{Total Time in Min}} \times \text{Drop Factor} = \text{Rate}$

   <u>Total volume</u> divided by <u>total time</u> in minutes, multiplied by the <u>drop factor calibration</u> in drops per milliliter, equals the flow <u>rate</u> in drops per minute.

   $\frac{\text{V}}{\text{T}} \times \text{C} = \text{R}$

2. $24\ h = 1440\ min$

   $\frac{\text{V}}{\text{T}} \times \text{C} = \text{R}$

   $\frac{3000\ \text{mL}}{1440\ \text{min}} \times \frac{10\ \text{gtt}}{\text{mL}} = 20.8 = \textbf{21 gtt/min}$

3. $5\ hr = 300\ min$

   $\frac{250\ \text{mL}}{300\ \text{min}} \times \frac{60\ \text{gtt}}{\text{mL}} = \textbf{50 gtt/min}$

4. $\frac{100\ \text{mL}}{40\ \text{min}} \times \frac{20\ \text{gtt}}{\text{mL}} = \textbf{50 gtt/min}$

5. $1\ hr = 60\ min$

   $\frac{25\ \text{mL}}{60\ \text{min}} \times \frac{60\ \text{gtt}}{\text{mL}} = \textbf{25 gtt/min}$

6. $4\ hr = 240\ min$

   Two 500 mL units of blood = 1000 mL total volume

   $\frac{1000\ \text{mL}}{240\ \text{min}} \times \frac{20\ \text{gtt}}{\text{mL}} = 83.3 = \textbf{83 gtt/min}$

7. $12\ h = 720\ min$

   $\frac{1240\ \text{mL}}{720\ \text{min}} \times \frac{20\ \text{gtt}}{\text{mL}} = 34.4 = \textbf{34 gtt/min}$

Review Set 35 (page 220)

1. **60** (minutes in one hour)

2. $\frac{60}{60} = \textbf{1}$

3. $\frac{60}{20} = \textbf{3}$

4. $\frac{60}{15} = \textbf{4}$

5. $\frac{60}{10} = \textbf{6}$

6. $\frac{\text{mL/h}}{\textbf{drop factor constant}} = \frac{\text{gtt}}{\text{min}}$

7. $\text{mL/h} = \frac{1000\ \text{mL}}{4\ \text{h}} = 250\ \text{mL/h}$

   $\frac{250}{4} = 62.5 = \textbf{63 gtt/min}$

8. $\text{mL/h} = \frac{750\ \text{mL}}{6\ \text{h}} = 125\ \text{mL/h}$

   $\frac{125}{3} = 41.66 = \textbf{42 gtt/min}$

9. $\text{mL/h} = \frac{500\ \text{mL}}{3\ \text{h}} = 166.7\ \text{mL/h} = 167\ \text{mL/h}$

   $\frac{167}{6} = 27.8 = \textbf{28 gtt/min}$

10. $\frac{60}{1} = \textbf{60 gtt/min}$

Review Set 36 (page 221)

1. $\frac{3000\ \text{mL}}{24\ \text{h}} = 125\ \text{mL/h}$

   $\frac{125\ \text{mL/h}}{4} = \textbf{31 gtt/min}$

2. $\frac{200\ \text{mL}}{2\ \text{h}} = 100\ \text{mL/h}$

   $\frac{100}{1} = \textbf{100 gtt/min}$

3. $\frac{800\ \text{mL}}{8\ \text{h}} = 100\ \text{mL/h}$

   $\frac{100}{3} = \textbf{33 gtt/min}$

4. $\frac{1000\ \text{mL}}{24\ \text{h}} = 42\ \text{mL/h}$

   $\frac{42}{1} = \textbf{42 gtt/min}$

5. $\frac{1500\ \text{mL}}{12\ \text{h}} = 125\ \text{mL/h}$

   $\frac{125}{4} = \textbf{31 gtt/min}$

6. $\frac{250\ \text{mL}}{2} = \textbf{125 mL/h}$

7. $\frac{2500\ \text{mL}}{24\ \text{h}} = 104\ \text{mL/h}$

   $\frac{104}{3} = \textbf{35 gtt/min}$

8. $\frac{500\ \text{mL}}{3\ \text{h}} = 166.7\ \text{mL/h} = 167\ \text{mL/h}$

   $\frac{167}{6} = \textbf{28 gtt/min}$

9. $\frac{1200 \text{ mL}}{8 \text{ h}} = 150 \text{ mL/h}$

   $\frac{150}{6} = \textbf{25 gtt/min}$

10. $\frac{1000 \text{ mL}}{8 \text{ h}} = \textbf{125 mL/h}$

11. $\frac{2000 \text{ mL}}{24 \text{ h}} = 83.3 = \textbf{83 mL/h}$

12. $\frac{500 \text{ mL}}{4 \text{ h}} = \textbf{125 mL/h}$

Review Set 37 (page 223)

1. $\frac{V}{T} \times C = R$

   $\frac{1500 \text{ mL}}{720 \text{ min}} \times \frac{20 \text{ gtt}}{\text{mL}} = 41.7 = \textbf{42 gtt/min}$

   After the sixth hour, 6 hours remain.

   $\frac{850}{360} \times 20 = 47.2 = 47 \text{ gtt/min}$

   Reset to 47 gtt/min (12% faster than original rate).

2. $\frac{V}{T} \times C = R$

   $\frac{1000 \text{ mL}}{360 \text{ min}} \times \frac{15 \text{ gtt}}{\text{mL}} = 41.7 = \textbf{42 gtt/min}$

   After 4 hours, 2 hours remain.

   $\frac{360}{120} \times 15 = 45 \text{ gtt/min}$

   Reset to 45 gtt/min (7% faster than original rate).

3. $\frac{V}{T} \times C = R$

   $\frac{1000 \text{ mL}}{480 \text{ min}} \times \frac{20 \text{ gtt}}{\text{mL}} = 41.7 = \textbf{42 gtt/min}$

   After 4 hours, 4 hours remain.

   $\frac{800}{240} \times 20 = 66.7 = 67 \text{ gtt/min (60\% faster)}$

   Ask my supervisor or the physician for a revised order, because the new rate would be 67 gtt/min (an increase of 60%).

4. $\frac{V}{T} \times C = R$

   $\frac{2000 \text{ mL}}{720 \text{ min}} \times \frac{10 \text{ gtt}}{\text{mL}} = 27.8 = \textbf{28 gtt/min}$

   After 8 hours, 4 hours remain.

   $\frac{750}{240} \times 10 = 31.3 = 31 \text{ gtt/min (11\% faster)}$

   Reset to 31 gtt/min.

5. $\frac{V}{T} \times C = R$

   $\frac{100 \text{ mL}}{240 \text{ min}} \times \frac{60 \text{ gtt}}{\text{mL}} = \textbf{25 gtt/min}$

   After 90 min, 150 min remain.

   $\frac{90}{150} \times 60 = 36 \text{ gtt/min (44\% faster)}$

   Ask my supervisor or the physician for a revised order, because the new rate would be 36 gtt/min (an increase of 44%).

Review Set 38 (page 225)

1. $\frac{V}{T} \times C = R$

   $\frac{100 \text{ mL}}{45 \text{ min}} \times \frac{60 \text{ gtt}}{\text{mL}} = 133.3 = \textbf{133 gtt/min}$

2. $\frac{100 \text{ mL}}{45 \text{ min}} = \frac{X \text{ mL}}{60 \text{ min}}$

   $45X = 6000$

   $\frac{45X}{45} = \frac{6000}{45}$

   $X = 133.3 = \textbf{133.3 mL/h}$

3. $\frac{V}{T} \times C = R$

   $\frac{50 \text{ mL}}{15 \text{ min}} \times \frac{15 \text{ gtt}}{\text{mL}} = \textbf{50 gtt/min}$

4. $\frac{50 \text{ mL}}{15 \text{ min}} = \frac{X \text{ mL}}{60 \text{ min}}$

   $15X = 3000$

   $\frac{15X}{15} = \frac{3000}{15}$

   $X = \textbf{200 mL/h}$

5. $\frac{V}{T} \times C = R$

   $\frac{50 \text{ mL}}{30 \text{ min}} \times \frac{60 \text{ gtt}}{\text{mL}} = \frac{50}{1} \times 2 = \textbf{100 gtt/min}$

Practice Problems—Chapter 11 (page 230)

1. $\frac{200 \text{ mL}}{120 \text{ min}} \times \frac{10 \text{ gtt}}{\text{mL}} = 16.7 = \textbf{17 gtt/min}$

2. $\frac{1000 \text{ mL}}{1440 \text{ min}} \times \frac{60 \text{ gtt}}{\text{mL}} = 41.7 = \textbf{42 gtt/min}$

3. $\frac{1500 \text{ mL}}{720 \text{ min}} \times \frac{20 \text{ gtt}}{\text{mL}} = 41.7 = \textbf{42 gtt/min}$

4. $\frac{200 \text{ mL}}{1440 \text{ min}} \times \frac{60 \text{ gtt}}{\text{mL}} = 8.3 = \textbf{8 gtt/min}$

5. $\frac{\text{Total mL}}{\text{Total hours}} = \frac{1000 \text{ mL}}{8 \text{ h}} = \textbf{125 mL/h}$

6. $\frac{800 \text{ mL}}{7 \text{ h}} = 114.28 = 114.3 \text{ mL/h}$

$\frac{114 - 125}{125} = -0.088 = -9\% \text{ decrease};$

within safe limits.

Assess patient. If stable, reset to 114 mL/h.

7. $\frac{3000 \text{ mL}}{1140 \text{ min}} \times \frac{15 \text{ gtt}}{\text{mL}} = \frac{45000}{1440} = 31.3 = \textbf{31 gtt/min}$

8. $\frac{125 \text{ mL}}{60 \text{ min}} \times \frac{20 \text{ gtt}}{\text{mL}} = 41.7 = \textbf{42 gtt/min}$

9. $\frac{1000 \text{ mL}}{360 \text{ min}} \times 15 \text{ gtt/mL} = \frac{15000}{360} = 41.67$

$= 42 \text{ gtt/min}$

$6 - 2 = 4 \text{ hours remaining}$

$\frac{800 \text{ mL}}{240 \text{ min}} \times 15 \text{ gtt/mL} = \frac{12000}{240} = 50 \text{ gtt/min}$

$50 - 42 = 8$

$\frac{50 - 42}{42} = \frac{8}{42} = 0.190 = 19\% \text{ increase}$

within safe limits of 25% variance.

Assess patient. If stable, reset to 50 gtt/min.

10. q.4h = 6 times/24 h = $6 \times 500 \text{ mL} = \textbf{3000 mL}$

11. **Abbott Laboratories**

12. **15 gtt/mL**

13. $\frac{60}{15} = \textbf{4}$

14. $\frac{500 \text{ mL}}{4 \text{ h}} = \textbf{125 mL/h}; \quad \frac{\text{mL/h}}{\text{drop factor constant}};$

$\frac{125 \text{ mL/h}}{4} = \textbf{31.25} = \textbf{31 gtt/min}$

15. $\frac{\text{V}}{\text{T}} \times \text{C} = \text{R}: \quad \frac{500 \text{ mL}}{240 \text{ min}} \times \frac{15 \text{ gtt}}{\text{mL}} = 31.25 = \textbf{31 gtt/min}$

16. 1530 + 4 h = 1530 + 0400 = 1930

1930 or 7:30 PM or 1900 − 1200 = 7:30 PM

17. $\frac{500 \text{ mL}}{4 \text{ h}} = \frac{X \text{ mL}}{2 \text{ h}}$

$4X = 1000$

$\frac{4X}{4} = \frac{1000}{4}$

$X = 250 \text{ mL}$

or, 500 mL/4 h = 125 mL/h

$\frac{125 \text{ mL}}{\text{h}} \times 2 \text{ h} = \textbf{250 mL}$

18. $\frac{210 \text{ mL}}{120 \text{ min}} \times 15 \text{ gtt/mL} = \frac{3150}{120} = 26.25 = 26 \text{ gtt/min}$

$\frac{26 - 31}{31} = -\frac{5}{31} = -0.161 = -16\% = \text{Decrease of 16\%};$

within safe limits.

Recalculate 210 mL to infuse over remaining 2 hours. Reset IV to 26 gtt/min.

19. $\frac{500 \text{ mL}}{4 \text{ h}} = \textbf{125 mL/h}$

20. $\frac{50 \text{ mL}}{30 \text{ min}} = \frac{X \text{ mL}}{60 \text{ min}}$

$30X = 3000$

$\frac{30X}{30} = \frac{3000}{30}$

$X = \textbf{100 mL/h}$

21. **Dextrose 2.5% in 0.45% sodium chloride.**

22. $5\% = 5 \text{ g dextrose per } 100 \text{ mL}$

$\frac{5 \text{ g}}{100 \text{ mL}} = \frac{X \text{ g}}{500 \text{ mL}}$

$100X = 2500$

$\frac{100X}{100} = \frac{2500}{100}$

$\textbf{X} = \textbf{25 g dextrose}$

$NS = 0.9 \text{ NaCl per } 100 \text{ mL}$

$\frac{0.9 \text{ g}}{100 \text{ mL}} = \frac{X \text{ g}}{500 \text{ mL}}$

$100X = 450$

$\frac{100X}{100} = \frac{450}{100}$

$\textbf{X} = \textbf{4.5 g NaCl}$

23. **A central line is a special catheter inserted to access a large vein in the chest.**

24. **A primary line is the IV tubing used to set up a primary IV infusion. It is long enough to reach from the IV bag to the hub of the IV catheter.**

25. **The purpose of a saline/heparin lock is to administer IV medications when the patient does not require IV fluids.**

26. **milliequivalent (mEq)**

27. **The purpose of the PCA pump is to allow the patient to self-administer IV medication for pain without having to call the nurse for a p.r.n. medication.**

28. **Advantages of the syringe pump are that a small amount of medication can be delivered directly from the syringe and a specified time can be programmed in the pump.**

29. **Phlebitis and infiltration.**

30. **Hourly (q.1h)**

31. **Blood loss occurring due to surgery, trauma, or hemorrhage; bone marrow depression in cancer patients, plasma clotting factors in hemophilia.**

32. **A, B, O, AB**

33. **At the bedside two nurses verify the identification band, blood bank number, blood type of donor, blood type of patient, donor number, ordered component, and expiration date of the blood. Both nurses sign the blood tag.**

34. **The Y-set system has two parts that allow normal saline to be infused to prime the IV line and ensure all of the blood is infused to the patient. The Y-set also contains a filter to remove debris or tiny clots.**

35. **Monitor for transfusion reactions.**

Review Set 39 (page 235)

1. $\frac{V}{T} \times C = R$

$$\frac{500 \text{ mL}}{T \text{ min}} \times \frac{20 \text{ gtt}}{1 \text{ mL}} = \frac{30 \text{ gtt}}{1 \text{ min}}$$

$$\frac{500}{T} \times \frac{20}{1} = \frac{30}{1}$$

$$\frac{10,000}{T} = \frac{30}{1}$$

$$30T = 10,000$$

$$\frac{30T}{30} = \frac{10,000}{30}$$

$$T = 333 \text{ min}$$

$$\frac{333 \text{ min}}{60} = \textbf{5 h 33 min or } 5\frac{1}{2} \textbf{ h}$$

2. $\frac{V}{T} \times C = R$

$$\frac{1000 \text{ mL}}{T} \times \frac{10 \text{ gtt}}{1 \text{ mL}} = \frac{25 \text{ gtt}}{1 \text{ min}}$$

$$\frac{10,000}{T} = \frac{25}{1}$$

$$25T = 10,000$$

$$\frac{25T}{25} = \frac{10,000}{25}$$

$$T = 400 \text{ min}$$

$$\frac{400 \text{ min}}{60} = \textbf{6 h 40 min} = 6\frac{2}{3} \textbf{ h}$$

3. $\frac{V}{T} \times C = R$

$$\frac{800 \text{ mL}}{T} \times \frac{15 \text{ gtt}}{1 \text{ mL}} = \frac{25 \text{ gtt}}{1 \text{ min}}$$

$$\frac{12,000}{T} = \frac{25}{1}$$

$$25T = 12,000$$

$$\frac{25T}{25} = \frac{12,000}{25}$$

$$T = 480 \text{ min}$$

$$\frac{480}{60} = \textbf{8 h}$$

4. Time : $\frac{20 \text{ mL}}{1 \text{ h}} = \frac{120 \text{ mL}}{X \text{ h}}$

$$20X = 120$$

$$\frac{20X}{20} = \frac{120}{60}$$

$$X = \textbf{6 h}$$

Rate : $\frac{\overset{1}{\cancel{120}} \text{ mL}}{\underset{3}{\cancel{360}} \text{ min}} \times \frac{60 \text{ gtt}}{1 \text{ mL}} = R$

$$R = \textbf{20 gtt/min}$$

5. Time : $\frac{20 \text{ mL}}{1 \text{ h}} = \frac{80 \text{ mL}}{X \text{ h}}$

$$20X = 80$$

$$\frac{20X}{20} = \frac{80}{20}$$

$$X = \textbf{4 h}$$

Rate : $\frac{80 \text{ mL}}{\underset{4}{\cancel{240}} \text{ min}} \times \frac{\overset{1}{\cancel{60}} \text{ gtt}}{1 \text{ mL}} = R$

$$R = \textbf{20 gtt/min}$$

6. $\frac{V}{T} \times C = R$

$$\frac{1200 \text{ mL}}{T} \times \frac{15 \text{ gtt}}{1 \text{ mL}} = \frac{27 \text{ gtt}}{1 \text{ min}}$$

$$\frac{18,000}{T} = \frac{27}{1}$$

$$27T = 18,000$$

$$\frac{27T}{27} = \frac{18,000}{27}$$

$$T = 667 \text{ min}$$

$$\frac{667 \text{ min}}{60} = 11 \text{ h } 7 \text{ min} = \textbf{about 11 h}$$

Completion time:

1600 + 1100 = 2700

2700 − 2400 = 0300

0300 or 3 AM the next morning.

7. Time : $\frac{125 \text{ mL}}{1 \text{ h}} = \frac{2000 \text{ mL}}{X \text{ h}}$

$$125X = 2000$$

$$\frac{125X}{125} = \frac{2000}{125}$$

$$X = 16 \text{ h}$$

Completion time:

$$1530 + 1600 = 3130$$

$$3130 - 2400 = 0730$$

0730 or 7:30 AM the next morning.

Rate : $\frac{2000 \text{ mL}}{960 \text{ min}} \times \frac{10 \text{ gtt}}{1 \text{ mL}} = R$

$$\frac{20,00\cancel{0}}{96\cancel{0}} = 20.8$$

$$R = \textbf{21 gtt/min}$$

8. $\dfrac{V}{T} \times C = R$

$$\dfrac{V}{1440 \text{ min}} \times \dfrac{60 \text{ gtt}}{1 \text{ mL}} = \dfrac{42 \text{ gtt}}{1 \text{ min}}$$

$$\dfrac{60V}{1440} = \dfrac{42}{1}$$

$$60V = 60480$$

$$\dfrac{60V}{60} = \dfrac{60480}{60}$$

$$V = 1008 \text{ mL}$$

1008 mL/24 h

9. $\dfrac{V}{T} \times C = R$

$$\dfrac{V}{1440 \text{ min}} \times \dfrac{15 \text{ gtt}}{1 \text{ mL}} = \dfrac{12 \text{ gtt}}{1 \text{ min}}$$

$$\dfrac{15V}{1440} = \dfrac{12}{1}$$

$$15V = 17280$$

$$\dfrac{15V}{15} = \dfrac{17280}{15}$$

$$V = 1152 \text{ mL}$$

1152 mL/24 h

10. $\dfrac{V}{1440 \text{ min}} \times \dfrac{10 \text{ gtt}}{1 \text{ mL}} = \dfrac{21 \text{ gtt}}{1 \text{ min}}$

$$\dfrac{10V}{1440} = \dfrac{21}{1}$$

$$10V = 30240$$

$$\dfrac{10V}{10} = 3024 \text{ mL}$$

3024 mL/24 h

Review Set 40 (page 238)

1. Total volume = 50 + 15 = **65 mL**

$$\dfrac{V}{T} \times C = \dfrac{65 \text{ mL}}{45 \text{ min}} \times 60 \text{ gtt/mL} = 86.66 = \textbf{87 gtt/min}$$

$$\dfrac{60 \text{ mg}}{2 \text{ mL}} = \dfrac{60 \text{ mg}}{X \text{ mL}}$$

$$60X = 120$$

$$\dfrac{60X}{60} = \dfrac{120}{60}$$

$$X = 2 \text{ mL antibiotic X}$$

Volume IV fluid to add to chamber = 50 − 2 = **48 mL**

2. Total volume = 60 + 15 = **75 mL**

$$\dfrac{V}{T} \times C = \dfrac{75 \text{ mL}}{60 \text{ min}} \times 60 \text{ gtt/mL} = \textbf{75 gtt/min}$$

$$\dfrac{75 \text{ mg}}{3 \text{ mL}} = \dfrac{75 \text{ mg}}{X \text{ mL}}$$

$$75X = 225$$

$$\dfrac{75X}{75} = \dfrac{225}{75}$$

$$X = 3 \text{ mL}$$

Volume IV fluid to add to chamber = 60 − 3 = **57 mL**

3. Total volume = 25 + 15 = **40 mL**

$$\dfrac{V}{T} \times C = \dfrac{40 \text{ mL}}{\overset{1}{\cancel{20}} \text{ min}} \times \overset{3}{\cancel{60}} \text{ gtt/mL} = \textbf{120 gtt/min}$$

$$\dfrac{15 \text{ mg}}{3 \text{ mL}} = \dfrac{15 \text{ mg}}{X \text{ mL}}$$

$$15X = 45$$

$$\dfrac{15X}{15} = \dfrac{45}{15}$$

$$X = 3 \text{ mL}$$

Volume IV fluid to add to chamber = 25 − 3 = **22 mL**

4. $\dfrac{50 \text{ mL}}{60 \text{ min}} = \dfrac{X \text{ mL}}{30 \text{ min}}$

$$60X = 1500$$

$$\dfrac{60X}{60} = \dfrac{1500}{60}$$

$$X = 25 \text{ mL total dilution volume}$$

$$\dfrac{125 \text{ mg}}{1 \text{ mL}} = \dfrac{250 \text{ mg}}{X \text{ mL}}$$

$$125X = 250$$

$$\dfrac{125X}{125} = \dfrac{250}{125}$$

$$X = 2 \text{ mL Ancef}$$

$$25 - 2 = 23 \text{ mL 0.9\% NaCl}$$

Add **23 mL** 0.9% NaCl and **2 mL** Ancef

5. $\dfrac{30 \text{ mL}}{60 \text{ min}} = \dfrac{X \text{ mL}}{20 \text{ min}}$

$$60X = 600$$

$$\dfrac{60X}{60} = \dfrac{600}{60}$$

$$X = 10 \text{ mL total dilution volume}$$

$$\dfrac{60 \text{ mg}}{2 \text{ mL}} = \dfrac{60 \text{ mg}}{X \text{ mL}}$$

$$60X = 120$$

$$\dfrac{60X}{60} = \dfrac{120}{60}$$

$$X = 2 \text{ mL Medication X}$$

Add **8 mL** D_5W and 2 mL Medication X.

Review Set 41 (page 240)

1. $\dfrac{20 \text{ mEq}}{1000 \text{ mL}} = \dfrac{X \text{ mEq}}{250 \text{ mL}}$

$$1000X = 5000$$

$$\dfrac{1000X}{1000} = \dfrac{5000}{1000}$$

$$X = \textbf{5 mEq} \text{ per 250 mL}$$

2. $\dfrac{2\ mEq}{1\ mL} = \dfrac{5\ mEq}{X\ mL}$

   $2X = 5$

   $\dfrac{2X}{2} = \dfrac{5}{2}$

   $X = \textbf{2.5 mL}$

3. The total volume is now 252.5 mL
   (250 mL D_5W + 2.5 mL KCl)

   $\dfrac{5\ mEq}{252.5\ mL} = \dfrac{X\ mEq}{15\ mL}$

   $252.5X = 75$

   $\dfrac{252.5X}{252.5} = \dfrac{75}{252.5}$

   $X = \textbf{0.297 mEq}$

   Child will receive 0.297 mEq/h or 0.3 mEq/h

4. $\dfrac{1000\ mg}{1000\ mL} = \dfrac{X\ mg}{250\ mL}$

   $1000X = 250000$

   $X = \textbf{250 mg}$

5. $\dfrac{500\ mg}{20\ mL} = \dfrac{250\ mg}{X\ mL}$

   $500X = 5000$

   $\dfrac{500X}{500} = \dfrac{5000}{500}$

   $X = \textbf{10 mL}$

   OR,

   $\dfrac{D}{H} \times Q = \dfrac{250\ mg}{500\ mg} \times 20\ mL = \textbf{10 mL}$

6. $\dfrac{250\ mg}{250\ mL} = \dfrac{X\ mg}{20\ mL}$

   $250X = 5000$

   $\dfrac{250X}{250} = \dfrac{5000}{250}$

   $X = 20\ mg$

   Child will receive 20 mg/h

7. 1 kg = 2.2 lb.

   $44\ lb = \dfrac{44}{2.2} = 20\ kg$

   $20\ kg \times 1\ mg/kg/h = \textbf{20 mg/h}$

8. **Yes**

Review Set 42 (page 243)

1. $\dfrac{100\ mg}{1\ mL} = \dfrac{400\ mg}{X\ mL}$

   $100X = 400$

   $\dfrac{100X}{100} = \dfrac{400}{100}$

   $X = \textbf{4 mL}$

2. $\dfrac{4\ mg}{1\ mL} = \dfrac{25\ mg}{X\ mL}$

   $4X = 25$

   $\dfrac{4X}{4} = \dfrac{25}{4}$

   $X = \textbf{6.3 mL}$

3. 25 kg child

   For the first 10 kg, at 100 mL/kg/day

   $\dfrac{100\ mL}{1\ kg} = \dfrac{X\ mL}{10\ kg}$

   $X = 1000\ mL$

   For the next 10 kg, at 50 mL/kg/day

   $\dfrac{50\ mL}{1\ kg} = \dfrac{X\ mL}{10\ kg}$

   $X = 500\ mL$

   25 kg − 20 kg = 5 kg remaining.

   For the last 5 kg, at 20 mL/kg/day

   $\dfrac{20\ mL}{1\ kg} = \dfrac{X\ mL}{5\ kg}$

   $X = 100\ mL$

   1000 mL + 500 mL + 100 mL = 1600 mL

   Total = 1600 mL/24 h

   $\dfrac{1600\ mL}{24\ h} = \textbf{66.7 or 67 mL/h}$

4. 13 kg child

   For the first 10 kg, at 100 mL/kg/day, as in #3

   $X = 1000\ mL$

   13 kg − 10 kg = 3 kg remaining.

   For the last 3 kg, at 50 mL/kg/day

   $\dfrac{50\ mL}{1\ kg} = \dfrac{X\ mL}{3\ kg}$

   $X = 150\ mL$

   1000 mL + 150 mL = 1150 mL

   Total = 1150 mL/24 h

   $\dfrac{1150\ mL}{24\ h} = 47.9 = \textbf{48 mL/h}$

Review Set 43 (page 246)

1. $\dfrac{25{,}000 \text{ U}}{1000 \text{ mL}} = \dfrac{1000 \text{ U/h}}{\text{X mL/h}}$

$25{,}000\text{X} = 1{,}000{,}000$

$\dfrac{25{,}000\text{X}}{25{,}000} = \dfrac{1{,}000{,}000}{25{,}000}$

$\text{X} = \textbf{40 mL/h}$

$\dfrac{\text{mL/h}}{\text{drop factor constant}} = \text{gtt / min}$

$\dfrac{40}{1} = \textbf{40 gtt/min}$

$\dfrac{1000 \text{ U}}{1 \text{ h}} = \dfrac{\text{X U}}{24 \text{ h}}$

$\text{X} = 24{,}000 \text{ U}$

Order is for 24,000 U/24 h.

Normal adult dosage = 20,000 – 40,000 U/day

Yes, it is safe.

2. $\dfrac{40{,}000 \text{ U}}{500 \text{ mL}} = \dfrac{1100 \text{ U/h}}{\text{X mL/h}}$

$40{,}000\text{X} = 550{,}000$

$\dfrac{40{,}000\text{X}}{40{,}000} = \dfrac{550{,}000}{40{,}000}$

$\text{X} = \textbf{14 mL/h}$

Yes, it is safe

$\dfrac{1100 \text{ U}}{1 \text{ h}} = \dfrac{\text{X U}}{24 \text{ h}}$

$\text{X} = 26{,}400 \text{ U}$

Order is for 26,400 U/24 h.

Yes, it is safe.

3. $\dfrac{25{,}000 \text{ U}}{500 \text{ mL}} = \dfrac{500 \text{ U/h}}{\text{X mL/h}}$

$25{,}000\text{X} = 250{,}000$

$\dfrac{25{,}000\text{X}}{25{,}000} = \dfrac{250{,}000}{25{,}000}$

$\text{X} = \textbf{10 mL/h}$

$\dfrac{\text{mL / h}}{\text{drop factor constant}} = \dfrac{10}{1} = \textbf{10 gtt/min}$

$\dfrac{500 \text{ U}}{1 \text{ h}} = \dfrac{\text{X U}}{24 \text{ h}}$

$\text{X} = 12{,}000 \text{ U}$

Order is for 12,000 U/24 h.

No, it is not safe.

4. $\dfrac{40{,}000 \text{ U}}{500 \text{ mL}} = \dfrac{2500 \text{ U/h}}{\text{X mL/h}}$

$40{,}000\text{X} = 1{,}250{,}000$

$\dfrac{40{,}000\text{X}}{40{,}000} = \dfrac{1{,}250{,}000}{40{,}000}$

$\text{X} = \textbf{31 mL/h}$

$\dfrac{2500 \text{ U}}{1 \text{ h}} = \dfrac{\text{X U}}{24 \text{ h}}$

$\text{X} = 60{,}000 \text{ U}$

Order is for 60,000 U/24 h.

Yes, the setting is accurate. Dosage is <u>not</u> safe. Contact the physician to review the order.

5. $\dfrac{25{,}000 \text{ U}}{1000 \text{ mL}} = \dfrac{\text{X U/h}}{120 \text{ mL/h}}$

$1000\text{X} = 3{,}000{,}000$

$\dfrac{1000\text{X}}{1000} = \dfrac{3{,}000{,}000}{1000}$

$\text{X} = 3000 \text{ U/h}$

$\dfrac{3000 \text{ U}}{1 \text{ h}} = \dfrac{\text{X U}}{24 \text{ h}}$

$\text{X} = 72{,}000 \text{ U}$

Order is for 72,000 U/24 h.

No, the dosage is not safe.

6. $\dfrac{30{,}000 \text{ U}}{500 \text{ mL}} = \dfrac{\text{X U/h}}{25 \text{ mL/h}}$

$500\text{X} = 750{,}000$

$\dfrac{500\text{X}}{500} = \dfrac{750{,}000}{500}$

$\text{X} = 1500 \text{ U/h}$

$\dfrac{1500 \text{ U}}{1 \text{ h}} = \dfrac{\text{X U}}{24 \text{ h}}$

$\text{X} = 36{,}000 \text{ U}$

Order is for 36,000 U/24 h.

Yes, the dosage is safe.

7. $\dfrac{40{,}000 \text{ U}}{1000 \text{ mL}} = \dfrac{\text{X U/h}}{80 \text{ mL/h}}$

$1000\text{X} = 3{,}200{,}000$

$\dfrac{1000\text{X}}{1000} = \dfrac{3{,}200{,}000}{1{,}000}$

$\text{X} = 3200 \text{ U/h}$

$\dfrac{3200 \text{ U}}{1 \text{ h}} = \dfrac{\text{X U}}{24 \text{ h}}$

$\text{X} = 76{,}800 \text{ U}$

Order is for 76,800 U/24 h.

No, the dosage is not safe.

8. $\dfrac{20,000 \text{ U}}{1000 \text{ mL}} = \dfrac{X \text{ U/h}}{60 \text{ mL/h}}$

$1000X = 1,200,000$

$\dfrac{1000X}{1000} = \dfrac{1,200,000}{1000}$

$X = 1200 \text{ U/h}$

$\dfrac{1200 \text{ U}}{1 \text{ h}} = \dfrac{X \text{ U}}{24 \text{ h}}$

$X = 28,800 \text{ U}$

Order is for 28,800 U/24 h.

Yes, the dosage is safe.

9. $\dfrac{30,000 \text{ U}}{500 \text{ mL}} = \dfrac{X \text{ U/h}}{96 \text{ mL/h}}$

$500X = 2,800,000 \text{ U}$

$\dfrac{500X}{500} = \dfrac{2,880,000}{500}$

$X = 5760 \text{ U/h}$

$\dfrac{5760 \text{ U}}{1 \text{ h}} = \dfrac{X \text{ U}}{24 \text{ h}}$

$X = 138,240 \text{ U}$

Order is for 138,240 U/24 h.

No, the dosage is not safe.

10. $\dfrac{10,000 \text{ U}}{1000 \text{ mL}} = \dfrac{X \text{ U/h}}{80 \text{ mL/h}}$

$1000X = 800,000$

$\dfrac{1,000X}{1,000} = \dfrac{800,000}{1,000}$

$X = 800 \text{ U/h}$

$\dfrac{800 \text{ U}}{1 \text{ h}} = \dfrac{X \text{ U}}{24 \text{ h}}$

$X = 19,200 \text{ U}$

Order is for 19,200 U/24 h.

No, the dosage is not safe.

11. $\dfrac{500 \text{ U}}{500 \text{ mL}} = \dfrac{10 \text{ U/h}}{X \text{ mL/h}}$

$500X = 5000$

$\dfrac{500X}{500} = \dfrac{5000}{500}$

$X = 10 \text{ mL/h}$

10 mL/h or 10 gtt/min

12. $\dfrac{40 \text{ mEq}}{1000 \text{ mL}} = \dfrac{2 \text{ mEq/h}}{X \text{ mL/h}}$

$40X = 2000$

$\dfrac{40X}{40} = \dfrac{2000}{40}$

$X = 50 \text{ mL/h}$

Review Set 44 (page 252)

1. 2 g = 2000 mg

$\dfrac{2000 \text{ mg}}{1000 \text{ mL}} = \dfrac{4 \text{ mg}}{X \text{ mL}}$

$2000X = 4000$

$\dfrac{2000X}{2000} = \dfrac{4000}{2000}$

$X = 2 \text{ mL}$

IV is to infuse at 2 mL/min

$\dfrac{2 \text{ mL}}{1 \text{ min}} = \dfrac{X \text{ mL}}{60 \text{ min}}$

$X = 120 \text{ mL}$

Rate is 120 mL/h

2. 0.5 g = 500 mg

$\dfrac{500 \text{ mg}}{250 \text{ mL}} = \dfrac{2 \text{ mg}}{X \text{ mL}}$

$500X = 500$

$\dfrac{500X}{500} = \dfrac{500}{500}$

$X = 1 \text{ mL}$

IV is to infuse at 1 mL/min

$\dfrac{1 \text{ mL}}{1 \text{ min}} = \dfrac{X \text{ mL}}{60 \text{ min}}$

$X = 60 \text{ mL}$

Rate is 60 mL/h

3. 2 mg = 2000 mcg

$\dfrac{2000 \text{ mcg}}{500 \text{ mL}} = \dfrac{5 \text{ mcg}}{X \text{ mL}}$

$2000X = 2500$

$\dfrac{2000X}{2000} = \dfrac{2500}{2000}$

$X = 1.25 \text{ mL}$

IV is to infuse at 1.25 mL/min

$\dfrac{1.25 \text{ mL}}{1 \text{ min}} = \dfrac{X \text{ mL}}{60 \text{ min}}$

$X = 75 \text{ mL}$

Rate is 75 mL/h

4. $198 \text{ lb} = \frac{198}{2.2} = 90 \text{ kg}$

per min,

$\frac{4 \text{ mcg}}{1 \text{ kg}} = \frac{X \text{ mcg}}{90 \text{ kg}}$

$\qquad X = 360 \text{ mcg}$

$360 \text{ mcg} = 360 \div 1000 = 0.36 \text{ mg}$

IV is to be set to provide 0.36 mg/min

$\frac{450 \text{ mg}}{500 \text{ mL}} = \frac{0.36 \text{ mg}}{X \text{ mL}}$

$450X = 180$

$\frac{450X}{450} = \frac{180}{450}$

$\qquad X = \frac{2}{5} = 0.4 \text{ mL}$

IV is to infuse at 0.4 mL/min

$\frac{0.4 \text{ mL}}{1 \text{ min}} = \frac{X \text{ mL}}{60 \text{ min}}$

$\qquad X = 24 \text{ mL}$

Rate is 24 mL/h

5. per minute, $\frac{15 \text{ mcg}}{1 \text{ kg}} = \frac{X \text{ mcg}}{70 \text{ kg}}$

$\qquad\qquad X = 1050 \text{ mcg}$

$1050 \text{ mcg} = 1050 \div 1000 = 1.05 \text{ mg}$

$\frac{800 \text{ mg}}{500 \text{ mL}} = \frac{1.05 \text{ mg}}{X \text{ mL}}$

$800X = 525$

$\frac{800X}{800} = \frac{525}{800}$

$\qquad X = 0.66 \text{ mL}$

IV is to infuse at 0.66 mL/min

$\frac{0.66 \text{ mL}}{1 \text{ min}} = \frac{X \text{ mL}}{60 \text{ min}}$

$\qquad X = 39.6 = 40 \text{ mL}$

Rate is 40 mL/h

6. $125 \text{ lbs} = \frac{125}{2.2} = 57 \text{ kg}$

per minute, minimum

$\frac{2.5 \text{ mcg}}{1 \text{ kg}} = \frac{X \text{ mcg}}{57 \text{ kg}}$

$\qquad X = 142.5 \text{ mcg}$

per minute, maximum

$\frac{10 \text{ mcg}}{1 \text{ kg}} = \frac{X \text{ mcg}}{57 \text{ kg}}$

$\qquad X = 570 \text{ mcg}$

Range is 142.5–570 mcg/min.

7. $142.5 \text{ mcg/min} - 570 \text{ mcg/min} = 0.1425 - 0.570 \text{ or}$

Range is 0.14–0.57 mg/min

8. $\frac{500 \text{ mg}}{500 \text{ mL}} = \frac{X \text{ mg}}{15 \text{ mL}}$

$500X = 7500$

$\frac{500X}{500} = \frac{7500}{500}$

$\qquad X = 15 \text{ mg}$

Rate is 15 mg/h.

$\frac{15 \text{ mg}}{60 \text{ min}} = \frac{X \text{ mg}}{1 \text{ min}}$

$60X = 15$

$\frac{60X}{60} = \frac{15}{60}$

$\qquad X = 0.25 \text{ mg}$

IV is delivering 0.25 mg/min.

Refer back to #7 range.

Yes, 0.25 mg/min is safe.

9. $2 \text{ g} = 2000 \text{ mg}$

$\frac{2000 \text{ mg}}{500 \text{ mL}} = \frac{X \text{ mg}}{60 \text{ mL}}$

$500X = 120,000$

$\frac{500X}{500} = \frac{120,000}{500}$

$\qquad X = 240 \text{ mg}$

IV is delivering 240 mg/h.

$\frac{240 \text{ mg}}{60 \text{ min}} = \frac{X \text{ mg}}{1 \text{ min}}$

$60X = 240$

$\frac{60X}{60} = \frac{240}{60}$

$\qquad X = 4 \text{ mg}$

IV is delivering 4 mg/min.

10. **Yes, 4 mg/min is within the normal range of 2–6 mg/min.**

11. Step 1: g/mL There are 20 g in 500 mL, how many mL are necessary to infuse 2 g?

$$\frac{20\ g}{500\ mL} = \frac{2\ g}{X\ mL}$$

$$20X = 1000$$

$$\frac{20X}{20} = \frac{100\cancel{0}}{2\cancel{0}}$$

$$X = 50\ mL$$

2 g are delivered by 50 mL.

Step 2: mL/h

What is the flow rate in mL/h to infuse 50 mL/30 min (which contains 2 g magnesium sulfate)?

$$\frac{50\ mL}{30\ min} = \frac{X\ mL}{60\ min}$$

$$30X = 3000$$

$$\frac{30X}{30} = \frac{300\cancel{0}}{3\cancel{0}}$$

$$X = \textbf{100 mL/h for bolus}$$

From the bolus calculation you know that 2 g = 50 mL.

$$\frac{2\ g}{50\ mL} = \frac{1\ g}{X\ mL}$$

$$2X = 50$$

$$\frac{2X}{2} = \frac{50}{2}$$

$$X = \textbf{25 mL/h for continuous infusion}$$

12. Step 1: U/mL (Equivalent: 1 U = 1000 mU, therefore, 1 mU = 0.001 U)

There are 15 U in 250 mL, how many mL are necessary to infuse 0.001 U (or 1 mU)?

$$\frac{15\ U}{250\ mL} = \frac{0.001\ U}{X\ mL}$$

$$15X = 0.25$$

$$\frac{15X}{15} = \frac{0.25}{15}$$

$$X = 0.02\ mL$$

Therefore 0.001 U or 1 mU = 0.02 mL

Step 2: mL/h

What is the flow rate in mL/h to infuse 0.02 mL/min (which contains 1 mU Pitocin)?

$$\frac{0.02\ mL}{1\ min} = \frac{X\ mL}{60\ min}$$

$$X = \textbf{1.2 mL}$$

Flow rate is 1 mL/h

Set the infusion pump at 1 mL/h to infuse the order of Pitocin of 1 mU/min.

Review Set 45 (page 254)

1. Step 1. IV PB Rate: $\frac{V}{T} \times C = R$

   $\frac{100 \text{ mL}}{30 \text{ min}} \times 10 \text{ gtt/mL} = \textbf{33 gtt/min}$

   Step 2. IV PB time: q.4h $\times$ 30 min = 6 $\times$ 30 = 180 min = 3 h

   Step 3. IV PB volume: 6 $\times$ 100 mL = 600 mL

   Step 4. Regular IV volume: 3000 mL – 600 mL = 2400 mL

   Step 5. Regular IV time: 24 h – 3 h = 21 h

   Step 6. Regular IV rate : $\frac{\text{mL/h}}{\text{drop factor constant}}$

   $\frac{2400 \text{ mL}}{21 \text{ h}} = 114 \text{ mL/h}$

   $\frac{114}{6} = \textbf{19 gtt/min}$

2. Step 1. IV PB rate: $\frac{V}{T} \times C = R$

   $\frac{40 \text{ mL}}{60 \text{ min}} \times 60 \text{ gtt/min} = \textbf{40 gtt/min}$

   Step 2. IV PB time: q.i.d. $\times$ 1 h = 4 times/day $\times$ 1 hour each time = 4 h per day

   Step 3. IV PB volume: 4 $\times$ 40 mL = 160 mL

   Step 4. Regular IV volume: 1000 mL – 160 mL = 840 mL

   Step 5. Regular IV time: 24 h – 4 h = 20 h = 1200 min

   Step 6. Regular IV rate: $\frac{V}{T} \times C = R$

   $\frac{840 \text{ mL}}{1200 \text{ min}} \times 60 \text{ gtt/mL} = \frac{840}{20} = \textbf{42 gtt/min}$

3. Step 1. IV PB rate: $\frac{50 \text{ mL}}{30 \text{ min}} \times 15 \text{ gtt/mL} = \textbf{25 gtt/min}$

   Step 2. IV PB time: q.6h $\times$ 30 min = 4 $\times$ 30 = 120 min = 2 h

   Step 3. IV PB volume: 4 $\times$ 50 = 200 mL

   Step 4. Reg. IV volume: 3000 mL – 200 mL = 2800 mL

   Step 5. Reg. IV time: 24 h – 2 h = 22 h

   Step 6. Reg. IV rate : $\frac{\text{mL/h}}{\text{drop factor constant}}$

   $\frac{2800 \text{ mL}}{22 \text{ h}} = 127 \text{ mL/h}$

   $\frac{127}{4} = 31.75 = \textbf{32 gtt/min}$

4. Step 1. IV PB rate: 50 mL/h $\times$ 1 h = **50 gtt/min**

   Step 2. IV PB time: q.6h = 4 times/day $\times$ 1 h/time = 4 h/day

   Step 3. IV PB volume: 50 $\times$ 4 = 200 mL

   Step 4. Reg. IV volume: 2000 mL – 200 mL = 1800 mL

   Step 5. Reg. IV time: 24 h – 4 h = 20 h

   Step 6. Reg. IV rate: $\frac{1800 \text{ mL}}{20 \text{ h}} = 90 \text{ mL/h} = \textbf{90 gtt/min}$

5. Step 1. IV PB rate: 50 mL/h = **50 gtt/min**

   Step 2. IV PB time: q.8h × 1 hour = 3 times/day × 1 h/time = 3 hours/day

   Step 3. IV PB volume: 50 × 3 = 150 mL

   Step 4. Reg. IV PB volume: 1000 mL − 150 mL = 850 mL

   Step 5. Reg. IV time: 24 h − 3 h = 21 h

   Step 6. Reg. IV rate: $\frac{850 \text{ mL}}{21 \text{ h}} = 40.48$ mL/h = **40 gtt/min**

6. Step 1. IV PB rate: $\frac{50 \text{ mL}}{30 \text{ min}} = \frac{X \text{ mL}}{60 \text{ min}}$

   $$30X = 3000$$

   $$\frac{30X}{30} = \frac{300\cancel{0}}{3\cancel{0}}$$

   $$X = 100 \text{ mL}$$

   Rate is 100 mL/h

   Step 2. IV PB time: q.6h × 30 min = $\frac{4 \text{ times}}{\text{day}} \times \frac{30 \text{ min}}{\text{time}} = \frac{120 \text{ min}}{\text{day}} = \frac{2 \text{ h}}{\text{day}}$

   Step 3. IV PB volume: 50 × 4 = 200 mL

   Step 4. Reg. IV volume: 2400 mL − 200 mL = 2200 mL

   Step 5. Reg. IV time: 24 h − 2 h = 22 h

   Step 6. Reg. IV rate: $\frac{2200 \text{ mL}}{22 \text{ h}} =$ **100 mL/h**

7. Step 1. IV PB rate: $\frac{100 \text{ mL}}{30 \text{ min}} = \frac{X \text{ mL}}{60 \text{ min}}$

   $$30X = 6000$$

   $$X = 200 \text{ mL}/60 \text{ min} = \textbf{200 mL/h}$$

   Step 2. IV PB time: q.8h × 30 min = $\frac{3 \text{ times}}{\text{day}} \times \frac{30 \text{ min}}{\text{time}} = 90 \text{ min} = 1\frac{1}{2}$ h

   Step 3. IV PB volume: 100 × 3 = 300 mL

   Step 4. Reg. IV volume: 2000 mL − 300 mL = 1700 mL

   Step 5. Reg. IV time: 24 h − $1\frac{1}{2}$ h = $22\frac{1}{2}$ h

   Step 6. Reg. IV rate: $\frac{1700}{22.5} = 75.56 =$ **76 mL/h**

8. Step 1. IV PB rate: $\frac{50 \text{ mL}}{15 \text{ min}} = \frac{X \text{ mL}}{60 \text{ min}}$

   $$15X = 3000$$

   $$\frac{15X}{15} = \frac{3000}{15}$$

   $$X = 200 \text{ mL}$$

   Rate is 200 mL/h

   Step 2. IV PB time: q.6h × 15 min = $\frac{4 \text{ times}}{\text{day}} \times \frac{15 \text{ min}}{\text{time}} = \frac{60 \text{ min}}{\text{day}} = \frac{1 \text{ h}}{\text{day}}$

   Step 3. IV PB volume: 50 × 4 = 200 mL

   Step 4. Reg. IV volume: 3000 mL − 200 mL = 2800 mL

   Step 5. Reg. IV time: 24 h − 1 h = 23

   Step 6. Reg. IV rate: $\frac{2800 \text{ mL}}{23 \text{ h}} = 121.74 =$ **122 mL/h**

Practice Problems—Chapter 12 (page 258)

1. Volume control sets are microdrip infusion sets **(60 gtt/mL).**

2. $\dfrac{1\,g}{5\,mL} = \dfrac{1\,g}{X\,mL}$

   $X = 5$ mL

   OR

   $\dfrac{D}{H} \times Q = \dfrac{1\,g}{1\,g} \times 5\,mL = \textbf{5 mL}$

3. $\dfrac{50\,mL}{60\,min} = \dfrac{X\,mL}{30\,min}$

   $60X = 1500$

   $\dfrac{60X}{60} = \dfrac{1500}{60}$

   $X = \textbf{25 mL total dilution volume}$

   $25\,mL - 5\,mL = \textbf{20 mL D}_5\textbf{W}$

4. $\dfrac{mL/h}{\text{drop factor constant}} = \dfrac{50}{1} = \textbf{50 gtt/min}$

5. **Once at 1200 h**

6. $\dfrac{25,000\,U/h}{250\,mL} = \dfrac{1200\,U}{X\,mL}$

   $25,000X = 300,000$

   $\dfrac{25,000X}{25,000} = \dfrac{300,000}{25,000}$

   $X = \textbf{12 mL/h}$

   $1200\,U/h \times 24\,h = 28,800\,U/24\,h$

   (Yes, it is within normal range of 20,000–40,000 U.)

7. $0.5\,g = 500\,mg$

   $\dfrac{500\,mg}{250\,mL} = \dfrac{30\,mg}{X\,mL}$

   $500X = 7500$

   $\dfrac{500X}{500} = \dfrac{7500}{500}$

   $X = \textbf{15 mL}$

   Rate is 15 mL/h

8. $\dfrac{20\,mEq}{1000\,mL} = \dfrac{X\,mEq}{250\,mL}$

   $1000X = 5000$

   $\dfrac{1000X}{1000} = \dfrac{5000}{1000}$

   $X = 5\,mEq$

   $\dfrac{2\,mEq}{1\,mL} = \dfrac{5\,mEq}{X\,mL}$

   $\dfrac{D}{H} \times Q = \dfrac{5\,mEq}{2\,mEq} \times 1\,mL = \textbf{2.5 mL}$

9. $2X = 5$

   $\dfrac{2X}{2} = \dfrac{5}{2}$

   $X = 2.5$ mL

   OR

   $\dfrac{40,000\,U}{1000\,mL} = \dfrac{X\,U/h}{100\,mL/h}$

   $1000X = 4,000,000$

   $\dfrac{1000X}{1000} = \dfrac{4,000,000}{1,000}$

   $X = \textbf{4000 U/h}$

   $4000\,U/h \times \dfrac{24\,h}{day} = 96,000\,U/day$

   No, it is not within normal range (20,000–40,000 U/day).

10. $1.5\,L = 1500\,mL$

    $\dfrac{4\,mL}{1\,min} = \dfrac{1500\,mL}{X\,min}$

    $4X = 1500$

    $\dfrac{4X}{4} = \dfrac{1500}{4}$

    $X = 375\,min$

    $\dfrac{375}{60} = 6\dfrac{15}{60} = 6\dfrac{1}{4}\,h = \textbf{6 h 15 min}$

11. $2\,g = 2000\,mg$

    $\dfrac{2000\,mg}{500\,mL} = \dfrac{4\,mg}{X\,mL}$

    $2000X = 2000$

    $\dfrac{2000X}{2000} = \dfrac{2000}{2000}$

    $X = 1\,mL$

    There are 4 mg Lidocane per 1 mL.

    IV must deliver 1 mL per min.

    $\dfrac{1\,mL}{1\,min} = \dfrac{X\,mL}{60\,min}$

    $X = 60\,mL$

    Rate must be 60 mL/h

12. $1\,g = 1000\,mg$

    $\dfrac{1000\,mg}{250\,mL} = \dfrac{3\,mg}{X\,mL}$

    $1000X = 750$

    $\dfrac{1000X}{1000} = \dfrac{750}{1000}$

    $X = 0.75\,mL$

    IV must deliver 0.75 mL/min to infuse 3 mg/min.

    $\dfrac{0.75\,mL}{1\,min} = \dfrac{X\,mL}{60\,min}$

    $X = 45\,mL$

    Rate = 45 mL/h

13. $1 \text{ g} = 1000 \text{ mg}$

$$\frac{1000 \text{ mg}}{500 \text{ mL}} = \frac{2 \text{ mg}}{X \text{ mL}}$$

$$1000X = 1000$$

$$\frac{1000X}{1000} = \frac{1000}{1000}$$

$$X = 1 \text{ mL}$$

IV must deliver 1 mL/min to infuse 2 mg/min.

$$\frac{1 \text{ mL}}{1 \text{ min}} = \frac{X \text{ mL}}{60 \text{ min}}$$

$$X = 60 \text{ mL}$$

Rate = **60 mL/h**

14. per minute,

$$80 \text{ kg} \times 50 \text{ mcg/kg} = 400 \text{ mcg}$$

$$400 \text{ mcg} = 400 \div 1000 = 0.4 \text{ mg}$$

$$\frac{250 \text{ mg}}{250 \text{ mL}} = \frac{0.4 \text{ mg}}{X \text{ mL}}$$

$$250X = 250 \times 0.4$$

$$\frac{250X}{250} = \frac{250 \times 0.4}{250}$$

$$X = 0.4 \text{ mL}$$

IV must deliver 0.4 mL/min to infuse 0.4 mg/min.

$$\frac{0.4 \text{ mL}}{1 \text{ min}} = \frac{X \text{ mL}}{60 \text{ min}}$$

$$X = 24 \text{ mL}$$

Rate = 24 mL/h

15. $2 \text{ g} = 2000 \text{ mg}$

$$\frac{2000 \text{ mg}}{1000 \text{ mL}} = \frac{X \text{ mg}}{75 \text{ mL}}$$

$$1000X = 150,000 \text{ mg}$$

$$\frac{1000X}{1000} = \frac{150,000}{1000}$$

$$X = 150 \text{ mg}$$

Patient is receiving 150 mg/h.

$$\frac{150 \text{ mg}}{60 \text{ min}} = \frac{X \text{ mg}}{1 \text{ min}}$$

$$60X = 150$$

$$\frac{60X}{60} = \frac{150}{60}$$

$$X = 2.5 \text{ mg}$$

IV is delivering 2.5 mg/min.

Yes, the range is 1–4 mg/min.

16. IV PB flow rate:

$$\frac{\text{mL/h}}{\text{drop factor constant}} = \frac{100 \text{ mL}}{6} = 16.67 = \textbf{17 gtt/min}$$

IV PB time:

q.6h × 1 h = 4 times/day × 1 hour/time = 4 hours/day

IV PB volume: 100 mL × 4 = 400 mL

Reg. IV volume: 3000 mL − 400 mL = 2600 mL

Reg. IV time: 24 h − 4 h = 20 h = 1200 min

Reg. IV rate:

$$\frac{2600 \text{ mL}}{20 \text{ h}} = 130 \text{ mL/h};$$

$$\frac{\text{mL/h}}{\text{drop factor constant}} = \frac{130 \text{ mL/h}}{6} = 21.67 = \textbf{22 gtt/min}$$

17. IV PB flow rate:

$$\frac{V}{T} \times C = R : \frac{50 \text{ mL}}{\overset{1}{\cancel{30}} \text{ min}} \times \overset{2}{\cancel{60}} \text{ gtt/mL} = \textbf{100 gtt/min}$$

IV PB time:

$$\text{q.i.d} \times 30 \text{ min} = \frac{4 \text{ times}}{\text{day}} \times \frac{30 \text{ min}}{\text{time}} = 120 \text{ min} = 2 \text{ h}$$

IV PB volume: 50 mL × 4 = 200 mL

Reg. IV volume: 3000 mL − 200 mL = 2800 mL

Reg. IV time: 24 h − 2 h = 22 h

Reg. IV rate:

$$\frac{V}{T} \times C = R \quad \frac{2800 \text{ mL}}{1320 \text{ min}} \times 60 \text{ gtt/mL} = \textbf{127 gtt/min}$$

18. $125 \text{ lb} = \frac{125}{2.2} = 57 \text{ kg}$

per minute,

$$57 \text{ kg} \times \frac{3 \text{ mcg}}{\text{kg}} = 171 \text{ mcg}$$

$$171 \text{ mcg} = 171 \div 1000 = 0.171 \text{ mg}$$

$$\frac{50 \text{ mg}}{500 \text{ mL}} = \frac{0.171 \text{ mg}}{X \text{ mL}}$$

$$50X = 85$$

$$\frac{50X}{50} = \frac{85}{50}$$

$$X = \frac{17}{10} = 1.7 \text{ mL}$$

IV must deliver 1.7 mL/min to infuse 171 mcg/min.

$$\frac{1.7 \text{ mL}}{1 \text{ min}} = \frac{X \text{ mL}}{60 \text{ min}}$$

$$X = 102 \text{ mL}$$

Rate = 120 mL/h

19. $1000 - 800 \text{ mL} = 200 \text{ mL infused}$

$$\frac{40 \text{ mEq}}{1000 \text{ mL}} = \frac{X \text{ mEq}}{200 \text{ mL}}$$

$$1000X = 8000$$

$$\frac{1000X}{1000} = \frac{8000}{1000}$$

$$X = \textbf{8 mEq}$$

20. $\frac{125 \text{ mL}}{60 \text{ min}} = \frac{X \text{ mL}}{1 \text{ min}}$

$$60X = 125$$

$$\frac{60X}{60} = \frac{125}{60}$$

$$X = \frac{25}{12} = 2\frac{1}{12} \text{ OR } \textbf{2 mL/min}$$

21. $\frac{V}{T} \times C = R$

$$\frac{250 \text{ mL}}{T} \times 10 \text{ gtt/mL} = 25 \text{ gtt/min}$$

$$\frac{2500}{T} = \frac{25}{1}$$

$$25T = 2500$$

$$\frac{25T}{25} = \frac{2500}{25}$$

$$T = 100 \text{ min} = \frac{100}{60} = \textbf{1 h 40 min}$$

22. $\frac{100 \text{ mL}}{T} \times 60 \text{ gtt/mL} = 33 \text{ gtt/min}$

$$\frac{6000}{T} = \frac{33}{1}$$

$$33\,T = 6000$$

$$\frac{33\,T}{33} = \frac{6000}{33}$$

$T = 181.82 = 182 \text{ min} = 3 \text{ h } \& \text{ 2 min} = 0302$

$1603 + 0302 = \textbf{1932 or 7:32 PM.}$

23. $\frac{V}{T} \times C = R$

$$\frac{V}{480 \text{ min}} \times 15 \text{ gtt/mL} = 48 \text{ gtt/min}$$

$$\frac{15\,V}{480} = \frac{48}{1}$$

$$\frac{15V}{15} = \frac{23,040}{15}$$

$$15V = 23,040$$

$$V = \textbf{1536 mL}$$

24. $\frac{100 \text{ mL}}{1 \text{ h}} = \frac{1500 \text{ mL}}{X \text{ h}}$

$$100X = 1500$$

$$\frac{100X}{100} = \frac{1500}{100}$$

$$X = \textbf{15 h}$$

25. $\frac{40 \text{ mEq}}{1000 \text{ mL}} = \frac{2 \text{ mEq/h}}{X \text{ mL/h}}$

$$40X = 2000$$

$$\frac{40X}{40} = \frac{2000}{40}$$

$$X = \textbf{50 mL/h = 50 gtt/min}$$

26. $75 \text{ mL/h} = \textbf{75 gtt/min}$

$$\frac{50,000 \text{ U}}{1000 \text{ mL}} = \frac{X \text{ U/h}}{75 \text{ mL/h}}$$

$$1000X = 3,750,000$$

$$\frac{1000X}{1000} = \frac{3,750,000}{1000}$$

$$X = 3750 \text{ U/h}$$

$3750 \text{ U/h} \times 24 \text{ h/day} = 90,000 \text{ U/day}$

No, the dosage is too high.

27. $\frac{5 \text{ mg}}{1 \text{ mL}} = \frac{37 \text{ mg}}{X \text{ mL}}$

$$5X = 37$$

$$\frac{5X}{5} = \frac{37}{5}$$

$$X = 7\frac{2}{5}$$

$$X = \textbf{7.4 mL}$$

28. per day, $\frac{100 \text{ mL}}{1 \text{ kg}} = \frac{X \text{ mL}}{8 \text{ kg}}$

$$X = 800 \text{ mL}$$

$$\frac{800 \text{ mL}}{24 \text{ h}} = \frac{X \text{ mL}}{1 \text{ h}}$$

$$24X = 800$$

$$\frac{24X}{24} = \frac{800}{24}$$

$$X = 33 \text{ mL/h}$$

$800 \div 24 = \textbf{33.3 or 33 mL/h}$

29. Step 1: g/mL

$$\frac{20 \text{ g}}{500 \text{ mL}} = \frac{3 \text{ g}}{\text{X mL}}$$

$$20X = 1500$$

$$\frac{20X}{20} = \frac{1500}{20}$$

$$X = 75 \text{ mL}$$

There are 3 g in 75 mL

Step 2: mL/h

$$\frac{75 \text{ mL}}{30 \text{ min}} = \frac{\text{X mL}}{60 \text{ min}}$$

$$30X = 4500$$

$$\frac{30X}{30} = \frac{4500}{30}$$

$$X = \textbf{150 mL/h for bolus infusion}$$

From bolus calculation you know there are 3 g in 75 mL

$$\frac{3 \text{ g}}{75 \text{ mL}} = \frac{2 \text{ g}}{\text{X mL}}$$

$$3X = 150$$

$$\frac{3X}{3} = \frac{150}{3}$$

$$X = \textbf{50 mL/h for continuous infusion of 2 g/h.}$$

30. Equivalent: 1 U = 1000 mU, therefore 1 mU = 0.001 U

Step 1: U/mL

There are 15 U in 500 mL, how many mL are necessary to infuse 0.001 U (or 1 mU)?

$$\frac{15 \text{ U}}{500 \text{ mL}} = \frac{0.0010}{\text{X mL}}$$

$$15X = 0.50$$

$$\frac{15X}{15} = \frac{0.50}{15}$$

$$X = 0.03 \text{ mL}$$

Therefore, 0.001 U or 1 mU = 0.03 mL

Step 2: mL/h

What is the flow rate in mL/h to infuse 0.03 mL/min (which contains 1 mU Pitocin)?

$$\frac{0.03 \text{ mL}}{1 \text{ min}} = \frac{\text{X mL}}{60 \text{ min}}$$

$$X = \textbf{1.8 rounded to 2 mL/h}$$

Part 2 Answers/Solutions to Posttest 1 and Posttest 2

(page 261)

1. O.U.

2. p.r.n

3. four times a day

4. hour of sleep (at bedtime)

5. intravenous piggyback

6. $°C = \dfrac{°F - 32}{1.8}$

   $°C = \dfrac{99 - 32}{1.8}$

   $°C = \dfrac{67}{1.8}$

   $°C = \mathbf{37.2°C}$

7. $°F = 1.8°C + 32$

   $°F = (1.8 \times 39°C) + 32$

   $°F = 70.2 + 32$

   $°F = \mathbf{102.2°F}$

8. $\dfrac{60 \text{ mg}}{1 \text{ tab}} = \dfrac{30 \text{ mg}}{X \text{ tab}}$

   $60X = 30$

   $\dfrac{60X}{60} = \dfrac{30}{60}$

   $X = \mathbf{\dfrac{1}{2} \text{ tablet}}$

9. $\dfrac{1 \text{ g}}{1000 \text{ mg}} = \dfrac{0.5 \text{ g}}{X \text{ mg}}$

   $X = 500 \text{ mg}$

   $\dfrac{500 \text{ mg}}{1 \text{ tab}} = \dfrac{250 \text{ mg}}{X \text{ tab}}$

   $500X = 250$

   $\dfrac{500X}{500} = \dfrac{250}{500}$

   $X = \mathbf{\dfrac{1}{2} \text{ tablet}}$

10. $\dfrac{1 \text{ mg}}{1000 \text{ mcg}} = \dfrac{0.3 \text{ mg}}{X \text{ mcg}}$

    $X = 300 \text{ mcg}$

    $\dfrac{150 \text{ mcg}}{1 \text{ tab}} = \dfrac{300 \text{ mcg}}{X \text{ tab}}$

    $150X = 300$

    $\dfrac{150X}{150} = \dfrac{300}{150}$

    $X = \mathbf{2 \text{ tablets}}$

11. $\dfrac{30 \text{ mg}}{1 \text{ tab}} = \dfrac{60 \text{ mg}}{X \text{ tab}}$

    $30X = 60$

    $\dfrac{30X}{30} = \dfrac{60}{30}$

    $X = \mathbf{2 \text{ tablets}}$

12. $\dfrac{400,000 \text{ U}}{5 \text{ mL}} = \dfrac{600,000 \text{ U}}{X \text{ mL}}$

    $400,000X = 3,000,000$

    $\dfrac{400,000X}{400,000} = \dfrac{3,000,000}{400,000}$

    $X = \mathbf{7.5 \text{ mL}}$

13. $\dfrac{1 \text{ g}}{1000 \text{ mg}} = \dfrac{0.6 \text{ g}}{X \text{ mg}}$

    $X = 600 \text{ mg}$

    $\dfrac{300 \text{ mg}}{1 \text{ cap}} = \dfrac{600 \text{ mg}}{X \text{ cap}}$

    $300X = 600$

    $\dfrac{300X}{300} = \dfrac{600}{300}$

    $X = \mathbf{2 \text{ capsules}}$

14. $\dfrac{\text{gr i}}{60 \text{ mg}} = \dfrac{\text{gr ss}}{X \text{ mg}}$

    $\dfrac{1}{60} = \dfrac{\frac{1}{2}}{X}$

    $X = \dfrac{1}{2} \times 60$

    $X = 30 \text{ mg}$

    $\dfrac{30 \text{ mg}}{1 \text{ tab}} = \dfrac{30 \text{ mg}}{X \text{ tab}}$

    $30X = 30$

    $\dfrac{30X}{30} = \dfrac{30}{30}$

    $X = \mathbf{1 \text{ tablet}}$

15. $\dfrac{\text{gr i}}{60 \text{ mg}} = \dfrac{\text{gr}\frac{1}{5}}{X \text{ mg}}$

$$\frac{1}{60} = \frac{\frac{1}{5}}{X}$$

$$X = \frac{1}{5} \times 60$$

$$X = 12 \text{ mg}$$

$$\frac{12 \text{ mg}}{1 \text{ tab}} = \frac{12 \text{ mg}}{X \text{ tab}}$$

$$12X = 12$$

$$\frac{12X}{12} = \frac{12}{12}$$

$$X = \textbf{1 tablet}$$

16. $\dfrac{250 \text{ mg}}{5 \text{ mL}} = \dfrac{175 \text{ mg}}{X \text{ mL}}$

$$250X = 875$$

$$\frac{250X}{250} = \frac{875}{250}$$

$$X = \textbf{3.5 mL}$$

17. $\dfrac{1 \text{ mg}}{1000 \text{ mcg}} = \dfrac{0.05 \text{ mg}}{X \text{ mcg}}$

$$X = 50 \text{ mcg}$$

$$\frac{50 \text{ mcg}}{1 \text{ tab}} = \frac{150 \text{ mcg}}{X \text{ tab}}$$

$$50X = 150$$

$$\frac{50X}{50} = \frac{150}{50}$$

$$X = \textbf{3 tablets}$$

18. $\dfrac{400 \text{ mg}}{5 \text{ mL}} = \dfrac{600 \text{ mg}}{X \text{ mL}}$

$$400X = 3000$$

$$\frac{400X}{400} = \frac{3000}{400}$$

$$X = \textbf{7.5 mL}$$

$$\frac{1 \text{ t}}{5 \text{ mL}} = \frac{X \text{ t}}{7.5 \text{ mL}}$$

$$5X = 7.5$$

$$\frac{5X}{5} = \frac{7.5}{5}$$

$$X = \textbf{1.5 t}$$

Give $1\frac{1}{2}$ t by mouth every six hours

19. $\dfrac{1 \text{ g}}{1000 \text{ mg}} = \dfrac{0.5 \text{ g}}{X \text{ mg}}$

$$X = 500 \text{ mg}$$

$$\frac{250 \text{ mg}}{1 \text{ tab}} = \frac{500 \text{ mg}}{X \text{ tab}}$$

$$250X = 500$$

$$\frac{250X}{250} = \frac{500}{250}$$

$$X = \textbf{2 tablets}$$

20. $\dfrac{\text{gr i}}{60 \text{ mg}} = \dfrac{\text{gr}\frac{1}{4}}{X \text{ mg}}$

$$X = \frac{1}{4} \times 60$$

$$X = 15 \text{ mg}$$

$$\frac{15 \text{ mg}}{1 \text{ mL}} = \frac{12 \text{ mg}}{X \text{ mL}}$$

$$15X = 12$$

$$\frac{15X}{15} = \frac{12}{15}$$

$$X = \frac{4}{5} = 0.8$$

$$X = \textbf{0.8 mL}$$

21. $\dfrac{\text{gr i}}{60 \text{ mg}} = \dfrac{\text{gr}\frac{1}{150}}{X \text{ mg}}$

$$X = \frac{1}{150} \times 60$$

$$X = \frac{6}{15} = \frac{2}{5} = 0.4$$

$$X = 0.4 \text{ mg}$$

$$\frac{0.4 \text{ mg}}{1 \text{ mL}} = \frac{0.4 \text{ mg}}{X \text{ mL}}$$

$$0.4X = 0.4$$

$$\frac{0.4X}{0.4} = \frac{0.4}{0.4}$$

$$X = \textbf{1 mL}$$

22. $\dfrac{75 \text{ mg}}{1.5 \text{ mL}} = \dfrac{65 \text{ mg}}{X \text{ mL}}$

$$75X = 97.5$$

$$\frac{75X}{75} = \frac{97.5}{75}$$

$$X = \textbf{1.3 mL}$$

23. $\dfrac{50 \text{ mg}}{1 \text{ mL}} = \dfrac{35 \text{ mg}}{X \text{ mL}}$

$$50X = 35$$

$$\frac{50X}{50} = \frac{35}{50}$$

$$X = \textbf{0.7 mL}$$

24. $\dfrac{100 \text{ mg}}{2 \text{ mL}} = \dfrac{25 \text{ mg}}{X \text{ mL}}$

$$100X = 50$$

$$\frac{100X}{100} = \frac{50}{100}$$

$$X = \textbf{0.5 mL}$$

25. $\dfrac{25 \text{ mg}}{1 \text{ mL}} = \dfrac{15 \text{ mg}}{X \text{ mL}}$

$$25X = 15$$

$$\frac{25X}{25} = \frac{15}{25}$$

$$X = \textbf{0.6 mL}$$

26. $\dfrac{1\text{ g}}{1000\text{ mg}} = \dfrac{0.3\text{ g}}{X\text{ mg}}$

    $X = 300\text{ mg}$

    $\dfrac{300\text{ mg}}{2\text{ mL}} = \dfrac{300\text{ mg}}{X\text{ mL}}$

    $300X = 600$

    $\dfrac{300X}{300} = \dfrac{600}{300}$

    $X = \textbf{2 mL}$

27. $\dfrac{1\text{ mg}}{1000\text{ mcg}} = \dfrac{0.5\text{ mg}}{X\text{ mcg}}$

    $X = 500\text{ mcg}$

    $\dfrac{1000\text{ mcg}}{1\text{ mL}} = \dfrac{500\text{ mcg}}{X\text{ mL}}$

    $1000X = 500$

    $\dfrac{1000X}{1000} = \dfrac{500}{1000}$

    $X = \textbf{0.5 mL}$

28. $\dfrac{40\text{ mg}}{1\text{ mL}} = \dfrac{50\text{ mg}}{X\text{ mL}}$

    $40X = 50$

    $\dfrac{40X}{40} = \dfrac{50}{40}$

    $X = 1\frac{1}{4} = 1.25$

    $X = \textbf{1.3 mL}$

29. $\dfrac{5\text{ mg}}{1\text{ mL}} = \dfrac{4\text{ mg}}{X\text{ mL}}$

    $5X = 4$

    $\dfrac{5X}{5} = \dfrac{4}{5}$

    $X = \textbf{0.8 mL}$

30. $\dfrac{10{,}000\text{ U}}{1\text{ mL}} = \dfrac{8000\text{ U}}{X\text{ mL}}$

    $10{,}000X = 8000$

    $\dfrac{10{,}000X}{10{,}000} = \dfrac{8000}{10{,}000}$

    $X = \textbf{0.8 mL}$

31. $\dfrac{25\text{ mg}}{0.5\text{ mL}} = \dfrac{20\text{ mg}}{X\text{ mL}}$

    $25X = 10$

    $\dfrac{25X}{25} = \dfrac{10}{25}$

    $X = \textbf{0.4 mL}$

32. $\dfrac{1\text{ g}}{3.7\text{ mL}} = \dfrac{1\text{ g}}{X\text{ mL}}$

    $X = \textbf{3.7 mL}$

    Divide this dose into two injections of 1.8 mL and 1.9 mL.

33. $\dfrac{1\text{ g}}{2.5\text{ mL}} = \dfrac{1.5\text{ g}}{X\text{ mL}}$

    $X = 3.75$

    $X = \textbf{3.8 mL}$

    Divide this dose into two injections of 1.9 mL each.

34. $1:5000 =$

    $\dfrac{1\text{ g}}{5000\text{ mL}} = \dfrac{1000\text{ mg}}{5000\text{ mL}} = \dfrac{1\text{ mg}}{5\text{ mL}}$

    $\dfrac{1\text{ mg}}{5\text{ mL}} = \dfrac{1\text{ mg}}{X\text{ mL}}$

    $X = \textbf{5 mL}$

35. $3000\text{ g} = 3000 \div 1000 = 3\text{ kg}$

    per day, $\dfrac{25\text{ mg}}{1\text{ kg}} = \dfrac{X\text{ mg}}{3\text{ kg}}$

    $X = 75\text{ mg}$

    75 mg divided q.i.d $= \dfrac{75}{4} = 18.75 = 19\text{ mg}$

36. $88\text{ lb} = \dfrac{88}{2.2} = 40\text{ kg}$

    $\dfrac{3\text{ mg}}{1\text{ kg}} = \dfrac{X\text{ mg}}{40\text{ kg}}$

    $X = 120\text{ mg}$

    $\dfrac{80\text{ mg}}{15\text{ mL}} = \dfrac{120\text{ mg}}{X\text{ mL}}$

    $80X = 1800$

    $\dfrac{80X}{80} = \dfrac{1800}{80}$

    $X = \textbf{22.5 mL}$

37. $20\text{ lb} = \dfrac{20}{2.2} = 9\text{ kg}$

    per day : $\dfrac{20\text{ mg}}{1\text{ kg}} = \dfrac{X\text{ mg}}{9\text{ kg}}$

    $X = 180\text{ mg}$

    per dose : $\dfrac{180\text{ mg}}{3\text{ doses}} = \dfrac{X\text{ mg}}{1\text{ dose}}$

    $3X = 180$

    $\dfrac{3X}{3} = \dfrac{180}{3}$

    $X = 60\text{ mg}$

    $\dfrac{125\text{ mg}}{5\text{ mL}} = \dfrac{60\text{ mg}}{X\text{ mL}}$

    $125X = 300$

    $\dfrac{125X}{125} = \dfrac{300}{125}$

    $X = 2.4\text{ mL}$

    $1\text{ t} = 5\text{ mL}$

    $\frac{1}{2}\text{ t} = 2.5\text{ mL}$ (is within 10% of 2.4 mL)

    Give $\frac{1}{2}$ t three times a day.

38. $\dfrac{2000 \text{ mL}}{24 \text{ h}} = 83.3 \text{ mL/h} = 83 \text{ mL/h}$

$\dfrac{\text{mL}/\text{h}}{\text{drop factor constant}} = \text{R}$

$\dfrac{83}{4} = 20.75 = \textbf{21 gtt/min}$

39. $\dfrac{10{,}000 \text{ U}}{500 \text{ mL}} = \dfrac{750 \text{ U}}{\text{X mL}}$

$10{,}000\text{X} = 375{,}000$

$\dfrac{10{,}000\text{X}}{10{,}000} = \dfrac{375{,}\cancel{000}}{10{,}\cancel{000}}$

$\qquad\quad \text{X} = 37.5 \text{ mL}$

750 U are in 37.5 mL

750 U/h = 750 U/38 mL

Flow rate = **38 mL/h**

40. $\qquad\qquad \dfrac{\text{V}}{\text{T}} \times \text{C} = \text{R}$

$\dfrac{400 \text{ mL}}{t} \times \dfrac{15 \text{ gtt}}{\text{mL}} = \dfrac{24 \text{ gtt}}{\text{min}}$

$\dfrac{400}{\text{T}} \times \dfrac{15}{1} = \dfrac{24}{1}$

$\dfrac{6000}{\text{T}} = \dfrac{24}{1}$

$24 \text{ T} = 6000$

$\dfrac{24 \text{ T}}{24} = \dfrac{6000}{24}$

$\text{T} = 250 \text{ min}$

$250 \text{ min} = \dfrac{250}{60} = 4 \text{ h } 10 \text{ min}$

$1530 + 0410 = \textbf{1940 or 7:40 PM}$

41. Step 1. IV PB rate: $\dfrac{\text{V}}{\text{T}} \times \text{C} = \text{R} \qquad \dfrac{100 \text{ mL}}{30 \text{ min}} \times 60 \text{ gtt/min} = \textbf{200 gtt/min}$ (IV PB rate)

Step 2. Total IV PB time: q.4h $\times$ 30 min = 6 $\times$ 30 = 180 min = 3 h

Step 3. Total volume of IV PB: 100 mL $\times$ 6 = 600 mL total

Step 4. Total volume of regular IV: 1500 mL – 600 mL = 900 mL

Step 5. Total regular time: 24 h – 3 h = 21 h

Step 6. Regular IV rate : $\dfrac{900 \text{ mL}}{21 \text{ h}} = 42.86 \text{ mL/h} = 43 \text{ mL/h}$

$\dfrac{\text{mL}/\text{h}}{\text{drop factor constant}} = \dfrac{43}{1} = \textbf{43 gtt/min}$ (Constant for 60 gtt/mL equals 1.)

42. $\dfrac{250{,}000 \text{ U}}{1 \text{ mL}} = \dfrac{300{,}000 \text{ U}}{\text{X mL}}$

$250{,}000\text{X} = 300{,}000$

$\dfrac{250{,}000\text{X}}{250{,}000} = \dfrac{300{,}\cancel{000}}{250{,}\cancel{000}}$

$\qquad\quad \text{X} = 1\tfrac{1}{5} = \textbf{1.2 mL}$

43.
$$8 \text{ h} \times \frac{60 \text{ min}}{\text{h}} = 480 \text{ min}$$

$$\frac{V}{T} \times C = R$$

$$\frac{V}{480 \text{ min}} \times 15 \text{ gtt/mL} = 32 \text{ gtt/min}$$

$$\frac{V}{480} \times \frac{15}{1} = \frac{32}{1}$$

$$\frac{15V}{480} = \frac{32}{1}$$

$$15V = 32 \times 480$$

$$15V = 15,360$$

$$\frac{15V}{15V} = \frac{15,360}{15}$$

$$V = \textbf{1024 mL}$$

44.
$$\frac{\text{gr i}}{60 \text{ mg}} = \frac{\text{gr}\frac{1}{8}}{X \text{ mg}}$$

$$X = \frac{1}{8} \times 60$$

$$X = 7.5 \text{ mg}$$

$$\frac{15 \text{ mg}}{1 \text{ mL}} = \frac{7.5 \text{ mg}}{X \text{ mL}}$$

$$15X = 7.5$$

$$\frac{15X}{15} = \frac{7.5}{15}$$

$$X = \textbf{0.5 mL}$$

or, computing using grains,

$$\frac{\text{gr}\frac{1}{4}}{1 \text{ mL}} = \frac{\text{gr}\frac{1}{8}}{X \text{ mL}}$$

$$\frac{1}{4}X = \frac{1}{8}$$

$$\frac{\frac{1}{4}X}{\frac{1}{4}} = \frac{\frac{1}{8}}{\frac{1}{4}}$$

$$X = \frac{1}{8} \times \frac{4}{1}$$

$$X = \textbf{0.5 mL}$$

45. 33 lb $= \frac{33}{2.2} = 15 \text{ kg}$

per day,
$$\frac{50 \text{ mg}}{1 \text{ kg}} = \frac{X \text{ mg}}{15 \text{ kg}}$$

$$X = 750 \text{ mg}$$

per q.12h dose,
$$\frac{750 \text{ mg}}{\text{day}} \div \frac{2 \text{ doses}}{\text{day}} = 375 \text{ mg/dose}$$

$$\frac{250 \text{ mg}}{5 \text{ mL}} = \frac{375 \text{ mg}}{X \text{ mL}}$$

$$250X = 1875$$

$$X = \frac{1875}{250}$$

$$X = \textbf{7.5 mL}$$

46.
$$\frac{500 \text{ mg}}{100 \text{ mL}} = \frac{250 \text{ mg}}{X \text{ mL}}$$

$$500X = 25000$$

$$\frac{500X}{500} = \frac{25000}{500}$$

$$X = \textbf{50 mL}$$

47.
$$\frac{10,000 \text{ U}}{1 \text{ mL}} = \frac{6000 \text{ U}}{X \text{ mL}}$$

$$10,000X = 6000$$

$$\frac{10,000X}{10,000} = \frac{6000}{10,000}$$

$$X = \textbf{0.6 mL}$$

48.
$$\frac{20 \text{ mEq}}{15 \text{ mL}} = \frac{20 \text{ mEq}}{X \text{ mL}}$$

$$20X = 300$$

$$\frac{20X}{20} = \frac{300}{20}$$

$$X = \textbf{15 mL}$$

49. From nomogram child's BSA = 0.8 m^2

$$\frac{2 \text{ mg}}{\text{m}^2} \times 0.8 \text{ m}^2 = 1.6 \text{ mg}$$

$$\frac{1 \text{ mg}}{1 \text{ mL}} = \frac{1.6 \text{ mg}}{X \text{ mL}}$$

$$X = \textbf{1.6 mL}$$

50. From nomogram child's BSA = 0.52 m^2

$$\frac{0.52 \text{ m}^2}{1.7 \text{ m}^2} \times 1000 \text{ mg} = \frac{520}{1.7} = 305.88 \text{ mg} = 306 \text{ mg}$$

$$\frac{500 \text{ mg}}{1 \text{ mL}} = \frac{306 \text{ mg}}{X \text{ mL}}$$

$$500X = 306$$

$$\frac{500X}{500} = \frac{306}{500}$$

$$X = 0.612$$

$$X = \textbf{0.61 mL}$$

51.
$$\frac{1 \text{ mg}}{1000 \text{ mcg}} = \frac{25 \text{ mg}}{X \text{ mcg}}$$

$$X = 25,000 \text{ mcg}$$

$$\frac{25,000 \text{ mcg}}{1,000 \text{ mL}} = \frac{5 \text{ mcg}}{X}$$

$$25,000X = 5,000$$

$$\frac{25,000X}{25,000} = \frac{5,000}{25,000}$$

$$X = 0.2 \text{ mL}$$

5 mcg/min will be infused by 0.2 mL/min

$$\frac{0.2 \text{ mL}}{1 \text{ min}} = \frac{X \text{ mL}}{60 \text{ min}}$$

$$X = 12 \text{ mL}$$

Rate is 12 mL/h

52. $\dfrac{40 \text{ mEq}}{1000 \text{ mL}} = \dfrac{2 \text{ mEq}}{X \text{ mL}}$

$40X = 2000$

$\dfrac{40X}{40} = \dfrac{200\cancel{0}}{4\cancel{0}}$

$X = 50 \text{ mL}$

2 mEq/h will be infused if rate is **50 mL/h** = 50 gtt/min

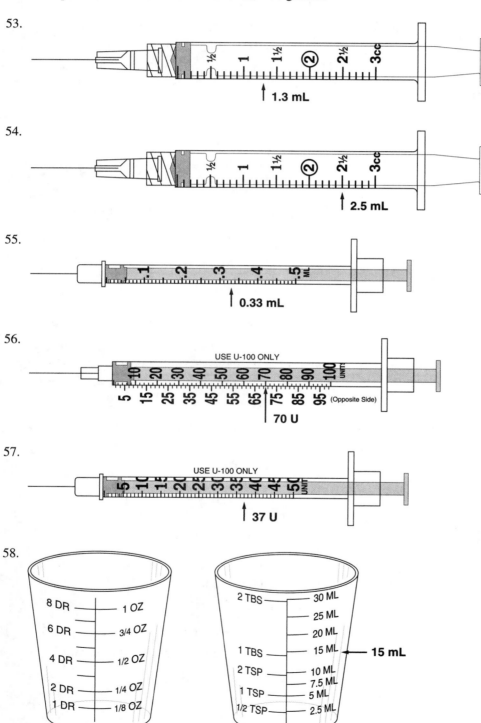

53.

  ↑ **1.3 mL**

54.

  ↑ **2.5 mL**

55.

  ↑ **0.33 mL**

56. USE U-100 ONLY

  (Opposite Side)

  ↑ **70 U**

57. USE U-100 ONLY

  ↑ **37 U**

58.

59.

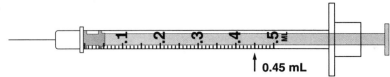

0.45 mL

60.

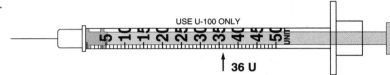

36 U

61. per day,

Minimum: $\dfrac{200 \text{ mg}}{1 \text{ kg}} = \dfrac{X \text{ mg}}{15 \text{ kg}}$

$\qquad X = 3000 \text{ mg}$

Maximum: $\dfrac{300 \text{ mg}}{1 \text{ kg}} = \dfrac{X \text{ mg}}{15 \text{ kg}}$

$\qquad X = 4500 \text{ mg}$

The 15 kg child could receive 3000–4500 mg/day.

62. $\dfrac{100 \text{ mg}}{1 \text{ mL}} = \dfrac{750 \text{ mg}}{X \text{ mL}}$

$\quad 100X = 750$

$\quad \dfrac{100X}{100} = \dfrac{75\cancel{0}}{10\cancel{0}}$

$\qquad X = \textbf{7.5 mL}$

63. **Dextrose 5% and normal saline (sodium chloride 0.9%) with 20 milliequivalents of potassium chloride per liter to run at a rate of 100 mL per hour.**

64. $\dfrac{20 \text{ mEq}}{1000 \text{ mL}} = \dfrac{X \text{ mEq}}{500 \text{ mL}}$

$\quad 1000X = 10,000$

$\quad \dfrac{1000X}{1000} = \dfrac{10\cancel{000}}{1\cancel{000}}$

$\qquad X = \textbf{10 mEq}$

65. $\dfrac{2 \text{ mEq}}{1 \text{ mL}} = \dfrac{10 \text{ mEq}}{X \text{ mL}}$

$\quad 2X = 10$

$\quad \dfrac{2X}{2} = \dfrac{10}{2}$

$\quad X = \textbf{5 mL}$

(page 267)

1. $\dfrac{10 \text{ mg}}{1 \text{ mL}} = \dfrac{20 \text{ mg}}{X \text{ mL}}$

    $10X = 20$

    $\dfrac{10X}{10} = \dfrac{20}{10}$

      $X = \textbf{2 mL}$

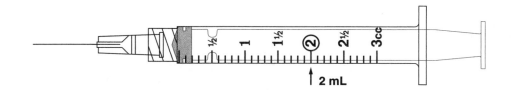

↑ **2 mL**

2. $\dfrac{20 \text{ mg}}{1 \text{ tab}} = \dfrac{20 \text{ mg}}{X \text{ tab}}$

    $20X = 20$

    $\dfrac{20X}{20} = \dfrac{20}{20}$

      $X = \textbf{1 tablet}$

3. $\dfrac{6.5 \text{ mg}}{1 \text{ cap}} = \dfrac{13 \text{ mg}}{X \text{ cap}}$

    $6.5X = 13$

    $\dfrac{6.5X}{6.5} = \dfrac{13}{6.5}$

      $X = \textbf{2 capsules}$

4. **SL = Sublingual.**

   (This means the medication is to be administered under the tongue.)

5. $\dfrac{0.25 \text{ mg}}{1 \text{ mL}} = \dfrac{0.25 \text{ mg}}{X \text{ mL}}$

    $0.25X = 0.25$

    $\dfrac{0.25X}{0.25} = \dfrac{0.25}{0.25}$

      $X = \textbf{1 mL stat, IV,}$
          repeated in 4 hours

$$0.5\overline{)0.25.} \quad \begin{array}{r} 0.5 \\ \hline \underline{25} \end{array}$$

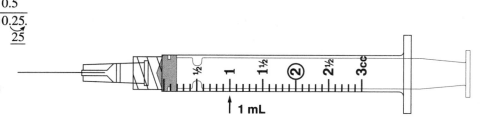

↑ **1 mL**

6. $\dfrac{0.25 \text{ mg}}{1 \text{ tab}} = \dfrac{0.125 \text{ mg}}{X \text{ tab}}$

    $0.25X = 0.125$

    $\dfrac{0.25X}{0.25} = \dfrac{0.125}{0.25}$

      $X = \dfrac{1}{2} \textbf{ tablet daily}$

$$0.25\overline{)0.125} \quad \begin{array}{r} 0.5 \\ \hline -125 \\ \hline 0 \end{array}$$

7. 80 mL/h (order)

   $\dfrac{V}{T} \times C = R$

   $\dfrac{80 \text{ mL/h}}{60 \text{ min}} \times 60 \text{ gtt/mL} = \textbf{80 gtt/min}$

8. $\dfrac{30 \text{ mEq}}{15 \text{ mL}} = \dfrac{10 \text{ mEq}}{X \text{ mL}}$

$30X = 150$

$\dfrac{30X}{30} = \dfrac{150}{30}$

$X = \textbf{5 mL}$

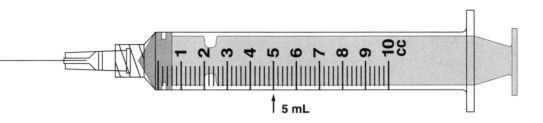

↑ **5 mL**

9. $\dfrac{10 \text{ mEq}}{1000 \text{ mL}} = \dfrac{X \text{ mEq/h}}{80 \text{ mL/h}}$

$1000X = 800$

$\dfrac{1000X}{1000} = \dfrac{800}{1000}$

$X = \textbf{0.8 mEq/h}$

10. $\dfrac{80 \text{ mL}}{1 \text{ h}} = \dfrac{X \text{ mL}}{24 \text{ h}}$

$X = \textbf{1920 mL}$

11. $\dfrac{80 \text{ mL}}{1 \text{ h}} = \dfrac{1000 \text{ mL}}{X \text{ h}}$

$80X = 1000$

$\dfrac{80X}{80} = \dfrac{1000}{80}$

$X = 12\frac{1}{2}$

Hang the next bag $12\frac{1}{2}$ hours after it is started.

$1630 + 1230 = 2900$

$2900 - 2400 = 0500$ or 5:30 AM the next morning, 9/4/XX

Hang new bag at 0500 on 9/4/XX

12. $\dfrac{325 \text{ mg}}{1 \text{ tab}} = \dfrac{650 \text{ mg}}{X \text{ tab}}$

$325X = 650$

$\dfrac{325X}{325} = \dfrac{650}{325}$

$X = \textbf{2 tablets}$

13. **80 mL/h**

14. **digoxin and acetaminophen**

15. $\dfrac{10 \text{ mg}}{1 \text{ mL}} = \dfrac{50 \text{ mg}}{X \text{ mL}}$

$10X = 50$

$\dfrac{10X}{10} = \dfrac{50}{10}$

$X = \textbf{5 mL}$

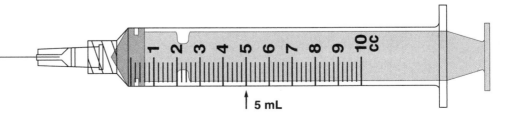

↑ **5 mL**

16. $\dfrac{2000\text{ mg}}{500\text{ mL}} = \dfrac{2\text{ mg}}{X\text{ mL}}$

$2000X = 1000$

$\dfrac{2000X}{2000} = \dfrac{1000}{2000}$

$X = 0.5\text{ mL}$

2 mg are in 0.5 mL; 2 mg/min requires 0.5 mL/min

$\dfrac{0.5\text{ mL}}{1\text{ min}} = \dfrac{X\text{ mL}}{60\text{ min}}$

$X = 30\text{ mL}$

Rate is 30 mL/h

17. $\dfrac{80\text{ mg}}{1\text{ mL}} = \dfrac{400\text{ mg}}{X\text{ mL}}$

$80X = 400$

$\dfrac{80X}{80} = \dfrac{400}{80}$

$X = \textbf{5 mL}$

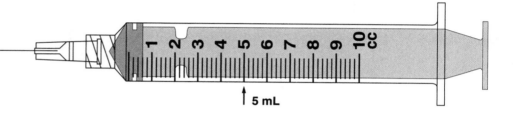

↑ **5 mL**

18. $110\text{ lb} = \dfrac{110}{2.2} = 50\text{ kg}$

per minute, $\quad \dfrac{10\text{ mcg}}{1\text{ kg}} = \dfrac{X\text{ mcg}}{50\text{ kg}}$

$X = 500\text{ mcg}$

$500\text{ mcg} = 500 \div 1000 = 0.5\text{ mg}$

$\dfrac{0.5\text{ mg}}{1\text{ min}} = \dfrac{X\text{ mg}}{60\text{ min}}$

$X = 30\text{ mg}$

Patient requires 30 mg per hour.

$\dfrac{400\text{ mg}}{250\text{ mL}} = \dfrac{30\text{ mg}}{X\text{ mL}}$

$400X = 7500$

$\dfrac{400X}{400} = \dfrac{7500}{400}$

$X = 18\dfrac{3}{4} = 18.75$

$X = 19\text{ mL}$

30 mg per hour would require a rate of **19 mL/h.**

19. $\dfrac{20\text{ mEq}}{1000\text{ mL}} = \dfrac{X\text{ mEq/h}}{50\text{ mL/h}}$

$1000X = 1000$

$\dfrac{1000X}{1000} = \dfrac{1000}{1000}$

$X = \textbf{1 mEq/h}$

20. In #16, it was computed that 2 mg/min required 30 mL/h so 4 mg/min requires 60 mL/h

OR,

$$\frac{2000 \text{ mg}}{500 \text{ mL}} = \frac{4 \text{ mg}}{X \text{ mL}}$$

$$2000X = 2000$$

$$\frac{2000X}{2000} = \frac{2000}{2000}$$

$$X = 1 \text{ mL}$$

4 mg are in 1 mL; 4 mg/min requires 1 mL/min

$$\frac{1 \text{ mL}}{1 \text{ min}} = \frac{X \text{ mL}}{60 \text{ min}}$$

$$X = 60 \text{ mL}$$

Rate is 60 mL/h

21. $$\frac{250 \text{ mg}}{5 \text{ mL}} = \frac{50 \text{ mg}}{X \text{ mL}}$$

$$250X = 250$$

$$\frac{250X}{250} = \frac{250}{250}$$

$$X = \textbf{1 mL}$$

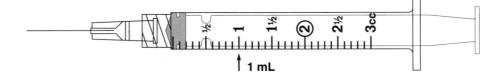

↑ **1 mL**

22. $$\frac{50 \text{ mg}}{1 \text{ mL}} = \frac{12.5 \text{ mg}}{X \text{ mL}}$$

$$50X = 12.5$$

$$\frac{50X}{50} = \frac{12.5}{50}$$

$$X = \textbf{0.25 mL}$$

↑ **0.25 mL**

23. $$\frac{25 \text{ mg}}{1 \text{ mL}} = \frac{35 \text{ mg}}{X \text{ mL}}$$

$$25X = 35$$

$$\frac{25X}{25} = \frac{35}{25}$$

$$X = \textbf{1.4 mL}$$

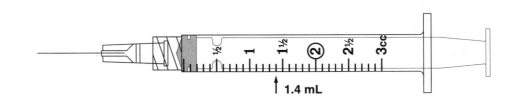

↑ **1.4 mL**

24. $$\frac{200 \text{ mg}}{1 \text{ tab}} = \frac{400 \text{ mg}}{X \text{ tab}}$$

$$200X = 400$$

$$\frac{200X}{200} = \frac{400}{200}$$

$$X = \textbf{2 tablets}$$

25. $$\frac{5 \text{ mg}}{1 \text{ tab}} = \frac{7.5 \text{ mg}}{X \text{ tab}}$$

$$5X = 7.5$$

$$\frac{5X}{5} = \frac{7.5}{5}$$

$$X = \mathbf{1\frac{1}{2} \text{ tablets}}$$

26. Reconstitute with **19 mL** diluent.

$$\frac{500 \text{ mg}}{100 \text{ mg}} \times 1 \text{ mL} = \textbf{5 mL} \text{ (see syringe)}$$

Add **5 mL** prostaphlin and **45 mL** D_5W to Buretrol (This will give a total of 50 mL to be infused.)

Flow rate: Total IV volume

$$\frac{V}{T} \times C = R$$

$$50 \text{ mL} + 15 \text{ mL flush} = 65 \text{ mL}$$

$$\frac{65 \text{ mL}}{60 \text{ min}} \times 60 \text{ gtt/mL} = \textbf{65 gtt/min}$$

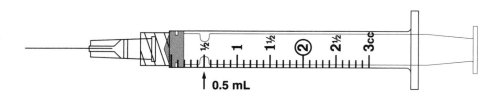

↑ **5 mL**

27. $$\frac{0.5 \text{ mg}}{2 \text{ mL}} = \frac{0.125 \text{ mg}}{X \text{ mL}}$$

$$0.5X = 0.250$$

$$\frac{0.5X}{0.5} = \frac{0.250}{0.5}$$

$$X = \textbf{0.5 mL}$$

↑ **0.5 mL**

28. $$\frac{\text{gr i}}{60 \text{ mg}} = \frac{\text{gr}\frac{1}{8}}{X \text{ mg}}$$

$$X = \frac{1}{8} \times 60$$

$$X = 7.5 \text{ mg}$$

$$\frac{15 \text{ mg}}{1 \text{ tab}} = \frac{7.5 \text{ mg}}{X \text{ tab}}$$

$$15X = 7.5$$

$$\frac{15X}{15} = \frac{7.5}{15}$$

$$X = \frac{1}{2} \textbf{ tablet}$$

29. $$\frac{500 \text{ mg}}{2 \text{ mL}} = \frac{350 \text{ mg}}{X \text{ mL}}$$

$$500X = 700$$

$$\frac{500X}{500} = \frac{700}{500}$$

$$X = \textbf{1.4 mL}$$

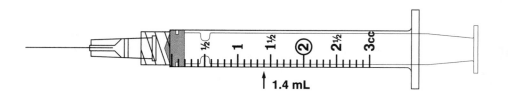

↑ **1.4 mL**

30. **Give 8 U, which equals 0.08 mL.**

$$\frac{100 \text{ U}}{1 \text{ mL}} = \frac{8 \text{ U}}{X \text{ mL}}$$

$$100X = 8$$

$$\frac{100X}{100} = \frac{8}{100}$$

$$X = \textbf{0.08 mL}$$

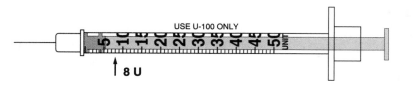

↑ **8 U**

31. $\dfrac{0.025 \text{ mg}}{1 \text{ tab}} = \dfrac{0.05 \text{ mg}}{X \text{ tab}}$

$0.025X = 0.05$

$\dfrac{0.025X}{0.025} = \dfrac{0.05}{0.025}$

$X = \textbf{2 tablets}$

32. $\dfrac{80 \text{ mg}}{1 \text{ tab}} = \dfrac{40 \text{ mg}}{X \text{ tab}}$

$80X = 40$

$\dfrac{80X}{80} = \dfrac{40}{80}$

$X = \dfrac{1}{2} \textbf{ tablet}$

33. $\dfrac{250 \text{ mg}}{1 \text{ tab}} = \dfrac{375 \text{ mg}}{X \text{ tab}}$

$250X = 375$

$\dfrac{250X}{250} = \dfrac{375}{250}$

$X = \mathbf{1\tfrac{1}{2} \textbf{ tablets}}$

34. $\dfrac{50 \text{ mg}}{1 \text{ mL}} = \dfrac{40 \text{ mg}}{X \text{ mL}}$

$50X = 40$

$\dfrac{50X}{50} = \dfrac{40}{50}$

$X = \textbf{0.8 mL}$

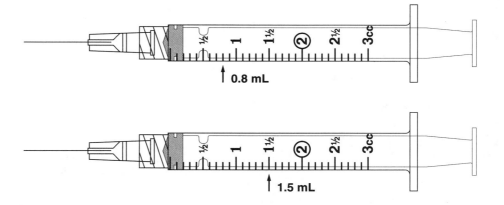

↑ 0.8 mL

35. $\dfrac{2 \text{ mg}}{1 \text{ mL}} = \dfrac{3 \text{ mg}}{X \text{ mL}}$

$2X = 3$

$\dfrac{2X}{2} = \dfrac{3}{2}$

$X = \textbf{1.5 mL}$

↑ 1.5 mL

36. $\dfrac{125 \text{ mg}}{5 \text{ mL}} = \dfrac{100 \text{ mg}}{X \text{ mL}}$

$125X = 500$

$\dfrac{125X}{125} = \dfrac{500}{125}$

$X = \textbf{4 mL}$

37. $\dfrac{\text{gr i}}{60 \text{ mg}} = \dfrac{\text{gr}\frac{1}{100}}{X \text{ mg}}$

$X = \dfrac{1}{100} \times 60$

$X = 0.6 \text{ mg}$

$\dfrac{0.4 \text{ mg}}{1 \text{ mL}} = \dfrac{0.6 \text{ mg}}{X \text{ mL}}$

$0.4X = 0.6$

$\dfrac{0.4X}{0.4} = \dfrac{0.6}{0.4}$

$X = \textbf{1.5 mL}$

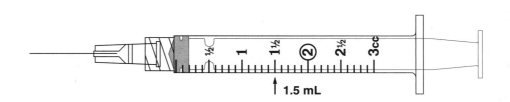

↑ 1.5 mL

38. $0.5 \text{ g} = 0.5 \times 1000 = 500 \text{ mg}$

$$\frac{250 \text{ mg}}{1 \text{ mL}} = \frac{500 \text{ mg}}{X \text{ mL}}$$

$$250X = 500$$

$$\frac{250X}{250} = \frac{500}{250}$$

$$X = \mathbf{2 \text{ mL}}$$

Add 2 mL Ampicillin to the normal saline.

Flow rate : $\frac{V}{T} \times C = R$

$$\frac{50 \text{ mL}}{30 \text{ min}} \times 15 \text{ gtt/mL} = \mathbf{25 \text{ gtt/min}}$$

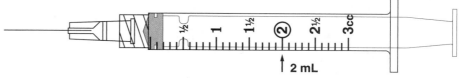

39. $\frac{5000 \text{ U}}{1 \text{ mL}} = \frac{10,000 \text{ U}}{X \text{ mL}}$

$$5000X = 10,000$$

$$\frac{5000X}{5000} = \frac{10,000}{5000}$$

$$X = \mathbf{2 \text{ mL}}$$

Add **2 mL** Heparin to IV solution.

$$\frac{10,000 \text{ U}}{500 \text{ mL}} = \frac{1200 \text{ U}}{X \text{ mL}}$$

$$10,000X = 600,000$$

$$\frac{10,000X}{10,000} = \frac{600,000}{10,000}$$

$$X = 60 \text{ mL}$$

Rate is 60 mL/h

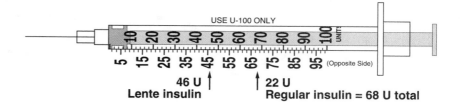

40. **Lente and regular insulin can be administered in the same syringe. Therefore, draw 22 units regular insulin in syringe and then draw 46 units Lente insulin for total of 68 units in your insulin syringe.**

41. $39°C \rightarrow °F$

$$°F = 1.8°C + 32$$
$$= (1.8 \times 39) + 32$$
$$= 70.2 + 32$$
$$= 102.2°F \text{ (This is greater than 101°F.)}$$

It has been 5 hours and 5 minutes since the last Tylenol was given; therefore, Tylenol may be given.

42. **2 tablets should be given for each dose.**

Each dose is equivalent to 650 mg Tylenol.

$$\frac{325 \text{ mg}}{1 \text{ tab}} = \frac{X \text{ mg}}{2 \text{ tab}}$$

$$X = \mathbf{650 \text{ mg}}$$

43. $\dfrac{60 \text{ mg}}{1 \text{ syringe}} = \dfrac{30 \text{ mg}}{X \text{ syringe}}$

$60X = 30$

$\dfrac{60X}{60} = \dfrac{30}{60}$

$X = \dfrac{1}{2}$

Give $\dfrac{1}{2}$ of the amount in the prefilled syringe.

44. **Select Nubain.**

$\dfrac{10 \text{ mg}}{1 \text{ mL}} = \dfrac{2 \text{ mg}}{X \text{ mL}}$

$10X = 2$

$\dfrac{10X}{10} = \dfrac{2}{10}$

$X = \textbf{0.2 mL}$

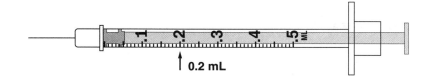

↑ **0.2 mL**

45. **Narcan**

$\dfrac{0.4 \text{ mg}}{1 \text{ mL}} = \dfrac{0.4 \text{ mg}}{X \text{ mL}}$

$0.4X = 0.4$

$\dfrac{0.4X}{0.4} = \dfrac{0.4}{0.4}$

$X = \textbf{1 mL}$

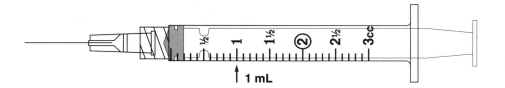

↑ **1 mL**

46. $\dfrac{250 \text{ mg}}{10 \text{ mL}} = \dfrac{150 \text{ mg}}{X \text{ mL}}$

$250X = 1500$

$\dfrac{250X}{250} = \dfrac{1500}{250}$

$X = 6 \text{ mL Aminophylline}$

50 mL total − 6 mL medication = 44 mL D_5W

$\dfrac{V}{T} \times C = R$

$\dfrac{50 \text{ mL}}{\overset{1}{\cancel{30}} \text{ min}} \times \dfrac{\overset{2}{\cancel{60}} \text{ gtt}}{\text{mL}} = \textbf{100 gtt/min}$

47. $\dfrac{50 \text{ mL}}{30 \text{ min}} = \dfrac{X \text{ mL}}{60 \text{ min}}$

$30X = 3000$

$\dfrac{30X}{30} = \dfrac{3000}{30}$

$X = \textbf{100 mL/h}$

OR, since using 60 gtt/mL infusion set, 100 gtt/min = 100 mL/h

48. **8 mL** diluent

$$\frac{62.5 \text{ mg}}{1 \text{ mL}} = \frac{125 \text{ mg}}{X \text{ mL}}$$

$$62.5X = 125$$

$$\frac{62.5X}{62.5} = \frac{125}{62.5}$$

$$X = \mathbf{2 \ mL}$$

OR

$$\frac{500 \text{ mg}}{8 \text{ mL}} = \frac{125 \text{ mg}}{X \text{ mL}}$$

$$500X = 1000$$

$$\frac{500X}{500} = \frac{1000}{500}$$

$$X = \mathbf{2 \ mL}$$

49. $\frac{D}{H} \times Q = \frac{1 \text{ g}}{1 \text{ g}} \times 1 \text{ tablet} = 1 \text{ tablet}$

Give 1 tablet at 0745, 1145, 1745, and 2145 hours.

50. **18 units**

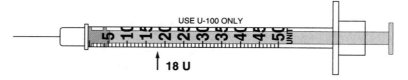

$\uparrow$ **18 U**

51. $32 \text{ lb} = \frac{32}{2.2} = 15 \text{ kg}$

per day, $\frac{15 \text{ mg}}{1 \text{ kg}} = \frac{X \text{ mg}}{15 \text{ kg}}$

$$X = 225 \text{ mg}$$

$$\frac{225 \text{ mg}}{3 \text{ doses}} = 75 \text{ mg/dose}$$

$$\frac{75 \text{ mg}}{2 \text{ mL}} = \frac{75 \text{ mg}}{X \text{ mL}}$$

$$75X = 150$$

$$\frac{75X}{75} = \frac{150}{75}$$

$$X = \mathbf{2 \ mL}$$

Buretrol = 60 gtt/min = C

25 mL solution + 15 mL flush = 40 mL total = V

$$\frac{V}{T} \times C = R$$

$$\frac{40 \text{ mL}}{60 \text{ min}} \times 60 \text{ gtt/mL} = 40 \text{ gtt/min}$$

Add **2 mL** Kantrex and **23 mL** D$_5$W to the Buretrol and set the flow rate for **40 gtt/min.**

52. $\frac{250 \text{ mg}}{250 \text{ mL}} = \frac{25 \text{ mg}}{X \text{ mL}}$

$$250X = 6250$$

$$\frac{250X}{250} = \frac{6250}{250}$$

$$X = 25 \text{ mL}$$

25 mg/h is infused by a rate of 25 mL/h

Rate = **25 mL/h**

53. $56 \text{ lb} = \frac{56}{2.2} = 25.4$ or 25 kg

    per hour, $\frac{1 \text{ mg}}{1 \text{ kg}} = \frac{X \text{ mg}}{25 \text{ kg}}$

    $X = 25$ mg

    Order is for 25 mg/h.

    Yes, the order is safe and reasonable.

54. Add **9 mL** water.

55. $15 \text{ lb} = \frac{15}{2.2} = 6.8$ or 7 kg

    Usual dose is 20 – 40 mg/kg/day

    in individual doses q.8h.

    per day,

    Minimum : $\frac{20 \text{ mg}}{1 \text{ kg}} = \frac{X \text{ mg}}{7 \text{ kg}}$ Maximum : $\frac{40 \text{ mg}}{1 \text{ kg}} = \frac{X \text{ mg}}{7 \text{ kg}}$

    $\quad\quad\quad\quad\quad X = 140$ mg $\quad\quad\quad\quad\quad\quad\quad X = 280$ mg

    $\frac{140 \text{ mg}}{3 \text{ doses}} = 46.6 = 47$ mg/dose

    $\frac{280}{3 \text{ doses}} = 93.3 = 93$ mg/dose

    Yes. The usual dosage is 20–40 mg/kg/day divided into 3 doses q.8h, which is equivalent to 47 mg–93 mg per dose for a 15-lb child.

56. $\frac{50 \text{ mg}}{1 \text{ mL}} = \frac{50 \text{ mg}}{X \text{ mL}}$

    $50X = 50$

    $\frac{50X}{50} = \frac{50}{50}$

    $X = \textbf{1 mL}$

57. (From label 50 mg = 1 dropperful)

    1 dropperful every 8 hours

58. $1 \text{ L} = 1000$ mL

    $\frac{20 \text{ mEq}}{1000 \text{ mL}} = \frac{X \text{ mEq}}{250 \text{ mL}}$

    $1000X = 5000$

    $\frac{1000X}{1000} = \frac{5000}{1000}$

    $X = \textbf{5 mEq}$

59. $\frac{2 \text{ mEq}}{1 \text{ mL}} = \frac{5 \text{ mEq}}{X \text{ mL}}$

    $2X = 5$

    $\frac{2X}{2} = \frac{5}{2}$

    $X = \textbf{2.5 mL}$

60. $110 \text{ lb} = \dfrac{110}{2.2} = 50 \text{ kg}$

$$\dfrac{5 \text{ mg}}{1 \text{ kg}} = \dfrac{X \text{ mg}}{50 \text{ kg}}$$

$$X = 250 \text{ mg}$$

$$\dfrac{300 \text{ mg}}{2 \text{ mL}} = \dfrac{250 \text{ mg}}{X \text{ mL}}$$

$$300X = 500$$

$$\dfrac{300X}{300} = \dfrac{500}{300}$$

$$X = \dfrac{5}{3} = 1\dfrac{2}{3} = 1.7 \text{ mL}$$

Add 1.7 mL of cimetidine.

$$\dfrac{V}{T} \times C = R$$

$$\dfrac{50 \text{ mL}}{\underset{2}{20} \text{ min}} \times \dfrac{\overset{1}{10} \text{ gtt}}{1 \text{ mL}} = \textbf{25 gtt/min}$$

61. $35 \text{ lb} = \dfrac{35}{2.2} = 15.9 \text{ or } 16 \text{ kg}$

$$\dfrac{20 \text{ mg}}{1 \text{ kg}} = \dfrac{X \text{ mg}}{16 \text{ kg}}$$

$$X = 320 \text{ mg}$$

$$\dfrac{500 \text{ mg}}{10 \text{ mL}} = \dfrac{320 \text{ mg}}{X \text{ mL}}$$

$$500X = 3200$$

$$\dfrac{500X}{500} = \dfrac{3200}{500}$$

$$X = \textbf{6.4 mL}$$

62. $50 \text{ mL} - 6.4 \text{ mL} = 43.6 \text{ mL} = \textbf{44 mL}$

63. $\dfrac{V}{T} \times C = R$

$$\dfrac{50 \text{ mL}}{60 \text{ min}} \times \dfrac{60 \text{ gtt}}{1 \text{ mL}} = \textbf{50 gtt/min}$$

64. $\dfrac{50 \text{ mL}}{60 \text{ min}} \times \dfrac{60 \text{ gtt}}{1 \text{ mL}} = \textbf{50 gtt/min}$

65. Jello : $\quad \dfrac{\text{Ʒ i}}{30 \text{ mL}} = \dfrac{\text{Ʒ 4}}{X \text{ mL}}$

$$X = 120 \text{ mL}$$

Water : $\quad \dfrac{\text{Ʒ 1}}{30 \text{ mL}} = \dfrac{\text{Ʒ 3}}{X \text{ mL}}$

$$X = 90 \text{ mL}$$

$$90 \text{ mL} \times 2 = 180 \text{ mL}$$

Juice : $\quad$ pt 1 = 500 mL

IV : $\quad \dfrac{50 \text{ mL}}{1 \text{ h}} = \dfrac{X \text{ mL}}{8 \text{ h}}$

$$X = 400 \text{ mL}$$

Total : $\quad$ 120

$\qquad\qquad$ 180

$\qquad\qquad$ 500

$\qquad \underline{+ \ 400}$ (Don't forget the IV fluids)

$\qquad \ \ \underline{\textbf{1200}}$ **mL**/8 h shift

Part 3   New Problems with Solutions

Chapter 2   Systems of Measurement

1. The abbreviation for milligram is _____.

2. The abbreviation for microgram is _____.

3. The abbreviation for kilogram is _____.

4. Identify the following basic liquid equivalents in the metric system:

   1 mL = _____cc

   1 L = _____ mL or _____ cc

5. The base unit used to measure length in the metric system is the _____.

6. List the five apothecary measurements of liquids.

   _____

   _____

   _____

   _____

   _____

7. Identify the following liquid equivalents:

   60 minims = _____

   8 fluidrams = _____

   32 fluidounces = _____

8. Interpret the following apothecary notations:

   ss _____

   iiiss _____

   gr _____

9. Express the following household measurements in proper notation.

   one tablespoon _____

   one quart _____

   one teaspoon _____

Interpret the following:

10. 20 mEq potassium chloride

11. Heparin 8000 U

Chapter 3   Conversions

1. Using the ratio-proportion method, convert each of the following amounts to the unit indicated. State the known equivalent.

   0.065 g = _____ mg

   500 cc = _____ L

2. The physician orders ferrous sulfate 600 mg orally. How many grains is this equivalent to? gr _____

3. You are to give phenobarbital 30 mg. You have phenobarbital 15 mg tablets. How many tablets will you give? _____ tablets

4. Convert 15 kg to pounds. _____ lb

5. Convert 4 t to milliliters. _____ mL

6. Convert 75 lb to kilograms. _____ kg

7. Milk of Magnesia ℥ ss is ordered. How many mL will you give? _____ mL

8. A patient receives ℥ i of fluid per hour from 0700–1500. How many mL will the patient receive in this period of time? _____ mL in _____ h

9. A patient will receive 1000 mL in 10 hours. How many mL/h will the patient receive? _____ mL in _____ h

10. The patient is to receive medication at 1300. This is equivalent to _____ o'clock (AM/PM)?

11. A patient has the following intake for breakfast. Calculate the intake in mL.

    milk _____ 8 oz

    orange juice _____ 4 oz

    coffee _____ 6 oz

12. A physician orders $1\frac{1}{2}$ t of medication. How many mL would you give?

Chapter 4   Equipment Used in Dosage Measurement

1. The nurse is to administer 3 mL of medication by the oral route. Which of the following devices could be utilized? (Place an X by the appropriate devices.)

   a. Medicine cup _____

   b. Syringe c̄ needle _____

   c. Calibrated dropper _____

   d. Syringe s̄ needle _____

   e. Prefilled, single-dose syringe _____

2. When using a U-100 Lo-Dose insulin syringe, 40 units of NPH insulin is equivalent to how many mL? _____

   a. 40 mL

   b. 0.04 mL

   c. 0.4 mL

   d. 4.0 mL

3. To administer 0.08 mL of medication intramuscularly, the nurse needs to use a _____.

   a. Carpuject cartridge-needle unit

   b. Tuberculin syringe

   c. Pre-filled, single-dose syringe

   d. 3 cc syringe

4. When measuring the correct dose for an intramuscular injection using a 3 cc syringe, the nurse reads the plunger at _____.

   a. The top black ring

   b. The raised middle section

   c. The bottom black ring

   d. Below the middle section

5. The medicine cup can measure all of the following *except* _____.

   a. ℥

   b. T

   c. mL

   d. m

6. An example of equipment for parenteral routes of administration is a _____.

   a. Tubex brand injection system

   b. Medicine cup

   c. Calibrated dropper

   d. 5 cc syringe s̄ needle

7. The nurse needs to administer 60 units of Lente Insulin. To administer the correct dosage of insulin the nurse needs to use a _____.

   a. U-100 Lo-Dose insulin syringe

   b Carpuject Cartridge

   c. U-100 100 U insulin syringe

   d. Tuberculin syringe

8. A calibrated dropper is used to administer which type of medication? _____

    a. Ear medications

    b. Insulin

    c. Parenteral medications

    d. Topical medications

9. When using a medicine cup for oral medication, 3 t is equivalent to _____.

    a. $\frac{1}{2}$ T

    b. 1 T

    c. 2 T

    d. 5 T

10. The nurse needs to administer 15 m of medication per injection. If the nurse uses a 3 cc syringe, at what cc mark will the top black ring of the plunger be positioned? _____

    Equivalent:

    60 m = 4 cc

    15 m = 1 cc

    a. 1 cc

    b. 1.5 cc

    c. 2 cc

    d. 2.5 cc

11. Which syringe is calibrated in tenths (0.1) of a cubic centimeter? _____

    a. U-100 insulin

    b. Tuberculin

    c. 3 cc

    d. U-100 Lo-Dose

12. Insulin syringes may be calibrated in either _____ unit or _____ units.

13. _____ syringes for injectable medications and _____ syringes for intravenous medications are utilized today to prevent needlestick injury.

Chapter 5   Interpreting Drug Orders

1. The physician orders Maalox 30 cc p.o. a.c. t.i.d. When would you give this medication? _____

    _____

2. Gentamycin opthalmic solution 2 gtt O.U. q.i.d. When and where would you administer this medication?

    _____

3. The physician orders Tylenol 325 mg p.o. stat and p.r.n., pain. When would you give this medication?

    _____

4. The physician orders ampicillin 1 gram IV PB q.8h. When and how would you administer this medication?

    _____

5. The physician orders Dalmane 15 mg p.o. h.s. When would you administer the Dalmane?

    _____

6. The physician orders Milk of Magnesia ℥ ii.

    a. How much of the medication would you administer? _____

    b. When would you administer the medication? _____

7. The physician orders Synthroid 25 mg p.o. q.d. How often would you administer this medication? _____

8. The physician orders Prednisone 10 mg p.o. q.i.d. × 5 days, 10 mg t.i.d. × 5 days, 10 mg b.i.d. × 5 days. How often would you administer this medication?

    _____

    _____

    _____

9. The physician orders Auralgen Otic Solution 1 gtt A.D. q.12h. Where and how often would you administer this medication?_____

10. Of the following medication orders, which one is incomplete? Why?

    Keflex 500 mg q.i.d.   gentamycin sulfate 50 mg IM q.8h

    _____

11. The physician writes the following medication orders:

    Multivitamin 1 tablet p.o. q.d.

    Digoxin 0.25 mg p.o. q.d.

    Lopressor 75 mg p.o. t.i.d.

    Dalmane 30 mg p.o. h.s.

    Kelflin 1 g IV PB 1.6h

    a. Which medication/s will the patient receive at regular intervals around the clock?

    _____

    b. Which medication/s will the patient receive one time, every day? _____

    c. When will the patient receive the Dalmane? _____

    d. How often will the patient receive the Lopressor? _____

12. A patient is receiving the following medications:

    Keflex 500 mg p.o. q.8h–0800–1600–2400

    Apresoline 25 mg p.o. b.i.d.–0800–2000

    Halcion 0.5 mg p.o. h.s.–2100

    If you are working the 7 A.M.–3 P.M. shift, which medications would you administer?

    _____

Chapter 6   Understanding Drug Labels

1. Information available on a drug label includes _____.
   a. Contraindications
   b. Side effects
   c. Expiration date
   d. Adverse reactions

2. An example of a generic name of a drug is _____.
   a. cephalexin capsules
   b. Lasix
   c. Geopen
   d. Dalmane

3. The expiration date on the drug ordered for the patient is September xxxx. Today is October 1, xxxx. The nurse should _____.
   a. Administer the medication
   b. Withhold the medication
   c. Substitute the medication
   d. Secure a fresh supply

4. The drug label indicates the medication on hand is an oral suspension. The nurse would expect to administer this drug by _____.
   a. Medicine cup
   b. Tuberculin syringe
   c. Topical application
   d. Sublingual

5. Given the following information, identify the response that indicates total volume of liquid in a vial of medication. _____
   a. 100 units per mL
   b. 20 mg/mL
   c. 10 mL vial
   d. 250 mg per 5 mL

6. The drug label reads that the medication can be administered IM/IV. The nurse should administer the medication _____.
   a. Parenterally
   b. Orally
   c. Rectally
   d. Topically

7. Dosage information on the drug label states ". . . usual adult dosage is 1 tablet every 4–6 hours . . ." The nurse understands that the patient should receive no more than _____ tablets in 24 hours.
   a. 4 tablets
   b. 6 tablets
   c. 12 tablets
   d. 8 tablets

8. The drug label reads Tylenol with Codeine tablets. The nurse interprets this drug label to mean that each dose of medication will include _____.

    a. 3 tablets

    b. 1 tablet of Tylenol; 3 tablets of Codeine

    c. $1\frac{1}{2}$ tablets of Tylenol; $1\frac{1}{2}$ tablets of Codeine

    d. A single tablet

9. The directions on the drug label indicate that the medication must be reconstituted. This means that the medication must be _____ before administration.

    a. mixed with diluent

    b. shaken well

    c. observed for precipitate

    d. refrigerated

10. The drug label on the medication bottle reads:

Russ®	Russ®
Lortab® 5 mg	100 Tablets
NDC 50474-902-60	Lortab® 5 mg

    This information indicates that _____.

    a. 100 tablets = 5 mg

    b. 60 tablets = 5 mg

    c. 1 tablet = 5 mg

    d. 1 dose = 500 mg

11. The purpose of the lot number is _____.

Chapter 7   Oral Dosage of Drugs

1. The physician orders digoxin 0.5 mg p.o. q.d. The medication available is digoxin 0.25 mg/10 mL. What is the quantity of medication to be administered? _____

2. The physician orders ampicillin 0.5 g p.o. q.6h. The medication is ampicillin 125 mg/5 mL. What is the quantity of medication to be administered? _____

3. The physician orders ASA gr viiss p.o. q.4h p.r.n. The medication available is ASA 300 mg per tablet. How many tablets will the nurse administer? _____

4. The physician orders morphine gr 1/4 p.o. q.6h p.r.n. The medication available is morphine 30 mg per tablet. How many tablets will the nurse administer? _____

5. The physician orders potassium chloride 50 mEq p.o. b.i.d. The medication available is potassium chloride 20 mEq/15 mL. How many mL will the nurse administer? _____

6. The physician orders Thyroid 100 mcg p.o. daily. The medication on hand is Thyroid 200 mcg per tablet. How many tablets will the nurse administer? _____

7. The physician orders amoxicillin 7.5 mL q.8h. The amoxicillin on hand is 125 mg per 5 mL.

    a. How many mg will the patient receive per dose? _____

    b. How many mg will the patient receive per day? _____

8. The physician orders Lanoxin 20 mcg p.o. q.d. The medication available is 0.04 mg per tablet. How many tablets will the nurse administer? _____

9. The physician orders Elixophyllin 120 mg p.o. q.6h. The medication available is Elixophyllin 80 mg/15 mL. How many mL will the patient receive per dose? _____

10. The Elixophyllin bottle contains ʒX. How many doses are available in ʒX for the order atropine gr 1/150 p.o. b.i.d.? _____

11. The physician orders atropine gr 1/150 p.o. b.i.d. The atropine available is 0.4 mg per tablet. The nurse will administer how many tablets per dose? _____

Interpret the following:

12. NG

13. NJ

14. GT

15. _____ medications and _____ tablets should not be crushed.

Chapter 8   Parenteral Dosage of Drugs

1. Physician orders Cleocin 0.5 g IM q.6h. The medication available Cleocin 300 mg/2 mL.

   Give _____.

2. The physician orders Lanoxin 0.09 mg IM STAT. The medication available Lanoxin 0.25 mg/mL.

   Give _____.

3. The physician orders gentamycin 10 mg IM b.i.d. The medication available gentamycin 40 mg/mL.

   Give _____.

4. The physician orders atropine gr 1/200 IM STAT. The medication available atropine 0.4 mg/mL.

   Give _____.

5. The physician orders Scopolamine g 1/400 IM q.d. The medication available is Scopolamine gr 1/150/cc.

   Give _____.

6. The physician orders 400,000 units of penicillin. The medication available is penicillin 1,000,000 U/cc in a 10 cc vial.

   a. How many cc will you administer? _____

   b. How many cc will be remaining in the vial? _____

7. The physician orders Rocephin 180 mg IM b.i.d. The medication available is Rocephin 1 g. Directions on the vial state "add 4.7 cc sterile water for injection to yield a concentration of 1 g/5 cc." After reconstitution, how many cc will you administer? _____

8. The physician orders ampicillin 750 mg IM b.i.d. The medication available is ampicillin 2 g. Directions on the vial state "dilute with 5 cc to yield 2 g/5.4 cc." After reconstitution, how many cc will you administer? _____

9. The physician orders 75 units of U-100 insulin. Only a tuberculin syringe is available. How many mL will you administer? _____

10. The physician orders adrenilin 0.5 mg IM STAT. The medication available is adrenilin 1:3000. How many mL will you administer? _____

11. The physician orders Lidocaine 50 mg for injection. The medication available is Lidocaine 20% solution. How many cc will you administer? _____

12. The physician orders magnesium sulfate 2 g for injection. The medication available is magnesium sulfate 50% solution. How many cc will you administer? _____

13. Explain the 70-30 concentration of insulin.

14. The physician orders 10 units of Regular insulin to be administered with 20 units of NPH insulin in the same syringe. Describe your actions step-by-step for mixing two types of insulin in the same syringe.

Chapter 9   Using the Formula Method to Calculate Dosages

1. The physician orders Tagamet 500 mg p.o. h.s. The medication available is Tagamet 200 mg/mL. Calculate the volume to be administered. _____

2. The physician orders glipizide 20 mg p.o. q A.M. The medication available is glipizide 5 mg scored tablets. How many tablets will you administer? _____

3. The physician orders ampicillin 0.4 g p.o. q.6h. The medication available is ampicillin oral suspension 250 mg/5 mL. How many mL will you administer? _____

4. The physician orders Apresoline 15 mg IM b.i.d. The medication available is Apresoline 20 mg/mL per ampule. How many mL will you administer? _____

5. The physician orders morphine 10 mg IM p.r.n. The medication available is morphine 15 mg/cc. How many cc of morphine will you administer? _____

6. The physician orders 60 mEq KCl to 1000 cc Lactated Ringers IV. The medication available is KCl 80 mEq/10 mL. How many mL of KCl will you add to the IV fluid? _____

7. The physician orders digoxin 0.25 mg IM STAT. The medication available is digoxin 0.1 mg/mL. How much digoxin will you administer? _____

8. The physician orders Lasix 40 mg p.o. b.i.d. The medication available is Lasix 10 mg/cc as an oral suspension. How much Lasix will you administer? _____

9. The physician orders Diabinese 500 mg p.o. every A.M. The medication available is Diaginese 250 mg/tablet. How many tablets will you administer? _____

10. The physician orders calcium gluconate 3 mEq to be added to 250 cc D_5W. The calcium gluconate available 0.45 mEq/mL. How many cc of calcium gluconate will be added to the IV fluid?

Chapter 10   Pediatric Dosages

Calculations for Oral Medication Administration

1. A doctor orders Amoxicillin Oral Suspension 100 mg p.o. q.8h. The infant weighs 10 kg. The recommended dose is 20–40 mg/kg/day in divided doses.

   a. Determine the safety of dosage. _____

   b. Amoxicillin available is 125 mg and needs to be reconstituted with 5 mL of water. Determine the quantity of medication to be administered. _____

2. A child weighs 48 lb and is to receive Slo-Phyllin 3 mg/kg q.6h. Slo-Phyllin available is 80 mg/15 mL. Determine the dosage and quantity to be administered. _____

3. An infant is to receive 30 mg of Tylenol for an elevated temperature. The recommended Tylenol dose is 10–15 mg/kg per dose. The Tylenol available is 80 mg/0.8 mL. The infant weights 3 kg. Determine the quantity to be administered. _____ Is the dosage safe?

4. A child weighs 15 kg and has a BSA of $0.6 m^2$. Secobarbital is ordered. The recommended dosage is 60 mg/m^2 t.i.d. Determine the dosage for this child. _____

5. A child weighs 40 kg and is 100 centimeters tall. The child is to receive Acyclovir. The recommended dosage is 250 mg/m. Calculate the correct dosage using the BSA method. _____

6. An infant has a BSA of $0.27 m^2$. The normal adult dose of Rocephin is 1 g daily in single or divided doses. Determine the dosage for this infant. _____

7. An 18-lb infant has a BSA of $0.38 m^2$. Ampicillin is ordered and the usual adult dose is 250 mg q.6h.

   a. Determine the dosage for this infant. _____

   b. The Ampicillin available is 250 mg/5 mL. Determine the quantity to be administered. _____

8. A child who weighs 50 lb and is normal height has digoxin ordered. The normal adult dosage is 0.25 mg.

   a. What is the child's dosage? _____

   b. The digoxin ampule contains 0.25 mg/cc. How many cc will you administer? _____

9. An infant weighs 4000 g. The physician orders Rocephin 250 mg IM daily divided in 2 equal doses. The recommended dosage is 50–100 mg/kg daily in 2 equal doses. Calculate the dosage range.

   a. Is the dosage safe? _____

   b. The Rocephin vial contains 1 g and is reconstituted with 3.6 mL diluent to yield 1 g/4 mL. How many mL will you administer in one dose? _____

10. The physician orders gentamycin 45 mg IM q.8h for a child who weighs 45 lb. The recommended dosage is 6–7.5 mg/kg daily in equal doses every 8 hours. Calculate the dosage range.

    a. Is the dose safe? _____

    b. The gentamycin vials available are 10 mg/mL and 40 mg/mL. Which one would you use? _____

    c. Calculate the amount of gentamycin you would administer. _____

11. The physician orders Acyclovir for a 12 kg child. The safe dosage of Acyclovir is 30 mg/kg/day given at 8 h intervals.

    a. What is the safe daily dosage for this child? _____

    b. What is the safe dose q.8h for this child? _____

12. The physician orders Septra IV for a child weighing 18 kg. The pediatric reference guide states that Septra is a combination medication containing 16 mg/mL of trimethroprim (TMP) and 80 mg/mL of sulfamethoxazole (SMZ). The safe dose of Septra is based on the TMP component and is recommended at a dosage range of 6–12 mg/kg/day of TMP divided q.12h.

   a. What dosage range of the TMP component should a child weighing 18 kg receive daily? _____

   b. What is the dosage range of TMP that the child should receive q.12h? _____

   c. If the physician ordered 6 mL of Septra IV q.12h for the 18 kg child, is the dosage safe?

Chapter 11   Intravenous Calculations

1. The physician orders 2 L $D_5 0.45\%$ NaCl IV in 24 hours by infusion pump. Calculate the flow rate. _____

2. The physician orders Rocephin 1 g IV in 100 cc NS IV PB in 45 minutes by infusion pump. Calculate the flow rate. _____

3. The physician orders 1600 cc D_5W IV in 18 hours by infusion pump. Calculate the flow rate. _____

4. Calculate the flow rate for 500 mL of $D_5 0.2\%$ NS IV to be infused in 8 hours. The drop factor is 20 gtt/mL. _____

5. Calculate the flow rate for 1000 cc Lactated Ringers IV to infuse in 10 hours. The drop factor is 15 gtt/mL. _____

6. Use the short-cut method to determine the IV flow rate in drops per minute. The physician orders 650 mL to infuse in 4 hours. The drop factor is 10 gtt/mL. _____

7. Use the short-cut method to determine the IV flow rate in drops per minute. The physician orders 1000 mL to infuse in 6 hours. The drop factor is 15 gtt/mL. _____

8. Use the short-cut method to determine the IV flow rate in drops per minute. The physician orders 850 mL to infuse in 8 hours. The drop factor is 60 gtt/mL. _____

9. The order reads 3000 mL D_5NS IV in 24 hours. The drop factor is 15 gtt/mL and the IV is correctly set at 31 gtt/min. After the seventh hour, you find 2500 cc remaining. Compute a new flow rate for the remaining 17 hours. _____ Is this rate reasonable?

10. Calculate the IV PB flow rate. The physician orders Mandol 2 g in 100 cc D_5W IV to be infused in 1 hour. The drop factor is 20 gtt/mL. _____

11. Calculate the IV PB flow rate. The physician orders ampicillin 500 mg in 50 cc NS IV to infuse in 40 minutes. The drop factor is 10 gtt/mL. _____

12. The physician orders Kefzol 1 g in 50 cc D_5W IV to infuse in 20 minutes. The drop factor is 15 gtt/mL.

    a. Calculate the IV PB flow rate. _____

    b. What is the flow rate if an infusion pump is used? _____

13. Calculate the amount of dextrose and sodium chloride in 250 mL of D_5NS.

Chapter 12   Advanced Intravenous Calculations

Calculate the IV flow rate to administer the following IV medications by Buretrol and determine the amount of IV fluid to be added to the Buretrol.

1. The physician orders cefuroxime sodium 3 g q.8h in 100 cc NS IV over 1 hour. Flush with 20 mL. The vial of cefuroxime sodium contains 1.5 g/5 mL.

    a. Total volume of cefuroxime sodium and flush: _____

    b. Flow rate of cefuroxime sodium and flush: _____

    c. Volume of cefuroxime sodium to be administered: _____

    d. Volume of IV fluid needed to be added to the Buretrol: _____

2. The physician orders ampicillin 150 mg in 50 cc D_5W followed by a 15 cc flush to infuse in 30 minutes. The ampicillin when reconstituted will yield 1 g/3 cc.

    a. Total volume of ampicillin and IV flush: _____

    b. Calculate the flow rate of the ampicillin and IV flush. _____

    c. Convert 1 g to mg. _____

    d. Volume of medication to be administered _____.

    e. Volume of IV fluid needed to be added to Buretrol for a solution of 50 cc: _____

3. The physician orders D_5W IV c̄ 40 mEq KCl/L to infuse at 25 mL/h.

    a. How many mEq of KCl will be added to a 500 cc bag? _____

    b. The KCl vial available is 80 mEq/10 cc. How many cc of KCl will be added to the 500 mL IV bag? _____

    c. How many mEq of KCl will the patient receive per hour? _____

4. The physician orders heparin IV 500 U/h. Determine the flow rate in mL/h and gtt/min if the heparin IV solution is 20,000 U in 250 cc NS. (Drop factor is 20 gtt/mL) _____

5. The physician orders 500 cc NS IV c̄ Heparin 30,000 U IV to infuse at 10 cc/h. What is the hourly dosage? _____

6. The physician orders lidocaine 100 mg IV in 50 cc D_5W to infuse at 4 mg/h. At what rate will you set the infusion pump? _____

7. The physician orders 2000 cc D_5NS IV to run at 65 cc/h. How long will this IV last? _____

8. Calculate the infusion time. The physician orders 150 mL NS IV at 30 gtt/min. The drop factor is 15 gtt/mL. _____

9. You start an IV infusion of Lactated Ringers at the rate of 40 gtt/min at 1500. The infusion set's drop factor is 10 gtt/mL. How much fluid will the patient receive in 12 hours? _____

10. The physician orders aminophylline 1 g in 100 mL NS IV at 23 mg/min. What rate will you set the infusion pump? _____

11. The physician orders 50 U Regular insulin in 100 mL NS IV. Administer 0.1 U/kg per minute. The patient weighs 75 lb. Determine the flow rate (mL/h).

    a. Desired dosage of medication: _____

    b. Determine the mL/min. _____

    c. Determine the flow rate. _____

12. The physician orders 1500 cc 0.45% NS for 24 h with gentamycin 40 mg/50 cc IV PB q.12h to run 1 hour. Limit total fluids to 1500 cc q.d. The drop factor is 15 gtt/mL. Calculate IV PB and IV rates.

   a. Flow rate of IV PB: _____

   b. Determine total time IV PB will be administered. _____

   c. Total volume of IV PB: _____

   d. Total volume IV fluids administered between IV PB per day: _____

   e. Total time of regular IV: _____

   f. Flow rate of regular IV: _____

13. If the minimum dilution for Solumedrol is 40 mg/mL and you are giving 30 mg, what is the least amount of fluid in which you could safely dilute the dose?

14. Calculate the hourly IV rate of a 22 kg child receiving maintenance IV fluids. You may use the following information for your calculations.

   1st 10 kg = 100 mL/kg/day

   2nd 10 kg = 50 mL/kg/day

   each additional kg = 20 mL/kg/day

Chapter 2   Systems of Measurement

1. mg

2. mcg

3. kg

4. 1 cc; 1000 ml or 1000 cc

5. meter

6. minim; pint; fluidram; quart; fluidounce

7. 1 fluidram; 1 fluidounce; 2 pints or 1 quart

8. $\frac{1}{2}$; $3\frac{1}{2}$; grain

9. 1 T;

   qt i

   1 t

10. 20 milliequivalents of potassium chloride

11. 8000 units of Heparin

Chapter 3   Conversion

1. **Known equivalent: 1 g = 1000 mg**

   $$\frac{1\text{ g}}{1000\text{ mg}} = \frac{0.065\text{ mg}}{X}$$
   $$X = 1000 \times 0.065 = 65\text{ mg}$$

   Known equivalent: 1 L = 1000 cc

   $$\frac{1\text{ L}}{1000\text{ cc}} = \frac{X}{500\text{ cc}}$$
   $$1000X = 500$$
   $$\frac{1000X}{1000} = \frac{500}{1000}$$
   $$X = 0.5\text{ L}$$

2. **Known equivalent: gr i = 60 mg**

   $$\frac{\text{gr i}}{60\text{ mg}} = \frac{X}{600\text{ mg}}$$
   $$60X = 300$$
   $$\frac{60X}{60} = \frac{300}{60}$$
   $$X = 10\text{ grams}$$
   $$= \text{gi X}$$

3. $$\frac{15\text{ mg}}{1\text{ tab}} = \frac{30\text{ mg}}{X\text{ tab}}$$
   $$15X = 30$$
   $$\frac{15X}{15} = \frac{30}{15}$$
   $$X = 2\text{ tablets}$$

4. $$\frac{1\text{ kg}}{2.2\text{ lb}} = \frac{15\text{ kg}}{X\text{ lb}}$$
   $$X = 33\text{ lb}$$

   Known equivalent: 1 kg = 2.2 lb

5. $$\frac{1\text{ t}}{5\text{ mL}} = \frac{4\text{ t}}{X\text{ mL}}$$
   $$X = 20\text{ mL}$$

6. $$\frac{1\text{ kg}}{2.2\text{ lb}} = \frac{X\text{ kg}}{75\text{ lb}}$$
   $$2.2X = 75$$
   $$\frac{2.2X}{2.2} = \frac{75}{2.2}$$
   $$X = 34\text{ kg}$$

   Known equivalent: 2.2 lb = 1 kg

7. **Known equivalent: ℥ = 30 mL**

   $$\frac{\text{℥ i}}{30\text{ mL}} = \frac{\text{℥ ss}}{X\text{ mL}}$$
   $$X = 30 \times \frac{1}{2}$$
   $$X = 15\text{ mL}$$

8. $$\text{℥ i} = 30\text{ mL}$$
   $$1500 - 0700 = 8\text{ h}$$
   $$30 \times 8 = 240\text{ mL in 8 hours}$$

9. $$\frac{1000\text{ mL}}{10\text{ h}} = \frac{100\text{ mL}}{1\text{ h}}$$

10. 1300 − 1200 = 1 h after noon = 1:00 PM

11. **Known equivalent 30 mL = 1 oz**

    $$8\text{ oz} + 4\text{ oz} + 6\text{ oz} = 18\text{ oz}$$
    $$\frac{\text{℥ i}}{30\text{ mL}} = \frac{\text{℥ 18}}{X\text{ mL}}$$
    $$X = 540\text{ mL}$$

12. **Known equivalent 5 mL = 1 tsp**

    $$\frac{5\text{ mL}}{1\text{ t}} = \frac{X\text{ mL}}{1\frac{1}{2}\text{ t}}$$
    $$X = 7.5\text{ mL}$$

Chapter 4   Equipment Used in Dosage Measurement

1. c, d

2. c

3. b

4. a

5. **d**

6. **a**

7. **c**

8. **a**

9. **b**

10. **a**

11. **c**

12. **1 unit or 2 units**

13. **Safety syringes; needleless syringes**

Chapter 5   Interpreting Drug Orders

1. **Before meals, three times a day, orally**

2. **Administer 2 drops in each eye, 4 times per day**

3. **Administer Tylenol immediately, by oral route and every 4 h when necessary for pain.**

4. **Administer 1 gram of ampicillin intravenous piggyback every 8 hours**

5. **Hour of sleep (at bedtime)**

6. a. **2 ounces**

   b. **When necessary**

7. **Once a day, every day**

8. **Administer Prednisone orally 4 times per day for 5 days; Administer Prednisone orally 3 times per day for 5 days; Administer Prednisone orally 2 times per day for 5 days**

9. **Administer 1 drop of Auralgen to right ear every 12 hours**

10. **Keflex order is incomplete. No route identified.**

11. a. **Keflin**

    b. **Multivitamin, Digoxin, and Dalmane**

    c. **Hour of sleep (at bedtime)**

    d. **Three times per day**

12. **Keflex and Apresoline**

Chapter 6   Understanding Drug Labels

1. **c**

2. **a**

3. **d**

4. **a**

5. **c**

6. **a**

7. **b**

8. **d**

9. **a**

10. **c**

11. **The purpose of the lot number is to identify the medication in case of a recall.**

Chapter 7   Oral Dosage of Drugs

1. $\dfrac{0.25 \text{ mg}}{10 \text{ mL}} = \dfrac{0.5 \text{ mg}}{X \text{ mL}}$

   $0.25X = 5$

   $\dfrac{0.25X}{0.25} = \dfrac{5}{0.25}$

   $X = 20 \text{ mL}$

2. **Equivalent: 1 g = 1000 mg**

   $\dfrac{1 \text{ g}}{1000 \text{ mg}} = \dfrac{0.5 \text{ g}}{X \text{ mg}}$

   $X = 500 \text{ mg}$

   $\dfrac{125 \text{ mg}}{5 \text{ mL}} = \dfrac{500 \text{ mg}}{X \text{ mL}}$

   $125X = 2500$

   $\dfrac{125X}{125} = \dfrac{2500}{125}$

   $X = 20 \text{ mL}$

3. **Equivalent: gr i = 60 mg**

   $\dfrac{\text{gr i}}{60 \text{ mg}} = \dfrac{\text{gr viiss}}{X \text{ mg}}$

   $\dfrac{1}{60} = \dfrac{7.5}{X}$

   $X = 450 \text{ mg}$

   $\dfrac{300 \text{ mg}}{1 \text{ tab}} = \dfrac{450 \text{ mg}}{X \text{ tab}}$

   $300X = 450$

   $\dfrac{300X}{300} = \dfrac{450}{300}$

   $X = 1\frac{1}{2} \text{ tablet}$

4. **Equivalent: gr i = 60 mg**

   $\dfrac{\text{gr i}}{60 \text{ mg}} = \dfrac{\text{gr}\frac{1}{4}}{X \text{ mg}}$

   $X = \dfrac{1}{4} \times 60$

   $X = 15 \text{ mg}$

   $\dfrac{30 \text{ mg}}{1 \text{ tab}} = \dfrac{15 \text{ mg}}{X \text{ tab}}$

   $30X = 15$

   $\dfrac{30X}{30} = \dfrac{15}{30}$

   $X = \dfrac{1}{2} \text{ tablet}$

5. $$\frac{20 \text{ mEq}}{15 \text{ mL}} = \frac{50 \text{ mEq}}{X \text{ mL}}$$

$$20X = 750$$

$$\frac{20X}{20} = \frac{750}{20}$$

$$X = 37.5 \text{ mL}$$

6. $$\frac{200 \text{ mcg}}{1 \text{ tab}} = \frac{100 \text{ mcg}}{X \text{ tab}}$$

$$200X = 100$$

$$\frac{200X}{200} = \frac{100}{200}$$

$$X = \frac{1}{2} \text{ tablet}$$

7. a. $$\frac{125 \text{ mg}}{5 \text{ mL}} = \frac{X \text{ mg}}{7.5 \text{ mL}}$$

$$5X = 937.5$$

$$\frac{5X}{5} = \frac{937.5}{5}$$

$$X = 187.5 \text{ or } 188 \text{ mg per dose}$$

  b. $$\frac{188 \text{ mg}}{1 \text{ dose}} = \frac{X \text{ mg}}{3 \text{ doses}}$$

$$X = 564 \text{ mg}$$

Patient will receive 564 mg/day.

8. $$\frac{1 \text{ mg}}{1000 \text{ mcg}} = \frac{0.04 \text{ mg}}{X \text{ mcg}}$$

$$X = 40 \text{ mcg}$$

$$\frac{40 \text{ mcg}}{1 \text{ tab}} = \frac{20 \text{ mcg}}{X \text{ tab}}$$

$$40X = 20$$

$$\frac{40X}{40} = \frac{20}{40}$$

$$X = \frac{1}{2} \text{ tablet}$$

9. $$\frac{80 \text{ mg}}{15 \text{ mL}} = \frac{120 \text{ mg}}{X \text{ mL}}$$

$$80X = 1800$$

$$\frac{80X}{80} = \frac{1800}{80}$$

$$X = 22.5 \text{ mL}$$

10. Equivalent: $\text{З i} = 30 \text{ mL}$

$$\frac{\text{З i}}{30 \text{ mL}} = \frac{\text{З X}}{X}$$

$$\frac{1}{30} = \frac{10}{X}$$

$$X = 300 \text{ mL}$$

$$22.5 \text{ mL} = 1 \text{ dose}$$

$$\frac{22.5 \text{ mL}}{1 \text{ dose}} = \frac{300 \text{ mL}}{X \text{ doses}}$$

$$22.5X = 300$$

$$\frac{22.5X}{22.5} = \frac{300}{22.5}$$

$$X = 13.3 \text{ or } 13 \text{ doses per bottle}$$

11. Equivalent: gr i = 60 mg

$$\frac{\text{gr i}}{60 \text{ mg}} = \frac{\text{gr} \frac{1}{150}}{X \text{ mg}}$$

$$X = \frac{1}{150} \times 60$$

$$X = 0.4 \text{ mg}$$

$$\frac{0.4 \text{ mg}}{1 \text{ tab}} = \frac{0.4 \text{ mg}}{X \text{ tab}}$$

$$0.4X = 0.4$$

$$\frac{0.4X}{0.4} = \frac{0.4}{0.4}$$

$$X = 1 \text{ tablet}$$

12. **NG = Nasogastric tube**

13. **NJ = Nasojejunal Tube**

14. **GT = Gastrostomy Tube**

15. **Enteric coated medications and sustained-release tablets should not be crushed.**

Chapter 8   Parenteral Dosage of Drugs

1. $$\frac{1 \text{ g}}{1000 \text{ mg}} = \frac{0.5 \text{ g}}{X \text{ mg}}$$

$$X = 500 \text{ mg}$$

$$\frac{300 \text{ mg}}{2 \text{ mL}} = \frac{500 \text{ mg}}{X \text{ mL}}$$

$$300X = 1000$$

$$\frac{300X}{300} = \frac{1000}{300}$$

$$X = 3.3 \text{ mL}$$

2. $$\frac{0.25 \text{ mg}}{1 \text{ mL}} = \frac{0.09 \text{ mg}}{X \text{ mL}}$$

$$0.25X = 0.09$$

$$\frac{0.25X}{0.25} = \frac{0.09}{0.25}$$

$$X = 0.36 \text{ mL}$$

3. $\frac{40 \text{ mg}}{1 \text{ mL}} = \frac{10 \text{ mg}}{X \text{ mL}}$

$40X = 10$

$\frac{40X}{40} = \frac{10}{40}$

$X = 0.25 \text{ mL}$

4. $\frac{\text{gr i}}{60 \text{ mg}} = \frac{\text{gr}\frac{1}{200}}{X \text{ mL}}$

$X = \frac{1}{200} \times 60$

$X = 0.3 \text{ mg}$

$\frac{0.4 \text{ mg}}{1 \text{ mL}} = \frac{0.3 \text{ mg}}{X \text{ mL}}$

$0.4X = 0.3$

$\frac{0.4X}{0.4} = \frac{0.3}{0.4}$

$X = 0.75 \text{ mL}$

5. $\frac{1}{150} = \frac{1}{400X}$

$\frac{400X}{400} = \frac{150}{400}$

$X = 3.75$

6. a. $\frac{1,000,000 \text{ U}}{1 \text{ cc}} = \frac{400,000 \text{ U}}{X \text{ cc}}$

$1,000,000X = 400,000$

$\frac{1,000,000X}{1,000,000} = \frac{400,000}{1,000,000}$

$X = 0.4 \text{ cc}$

b. $\begin{array}{r} 10.0 \\ - 0.4 \\ \hline 9.6 \text{ cc remaining in the vial} \end{array}$

7. $1 \text{ g} = 1000 \text{ mg}$

$\frac{1000 \text{ mg}}{5 \text{ cc}} = \frac{180 \text{ mg}}{X \text{ cc}}$

$1000X = 900$

$\frac{1000X}{1000} = \frac{900}{1000}$

$X = 0.9 \text{ cc}$

8. **Convert g to mg. Equivalent: 1 g = 1000 mg**

$2 \text{ g} = 2000 \text{ mg}$

$\frac{2000 \text{ mg}}{5.4 \text{ cc}} = \frac{750 \text{ mg}}{X \text{ cc}}$

$2000X = 4050$

$\frac{2000X}{2000} = \frac{4050}{2000}$

$X = 2.025$

$X = 2.0 \text{ cc}$

9. **U-100 insulin, 100 U = 1 mL**

$\frac{100 \text{ U}}{1 \text{ mL}} = \frac{75 \text{ U}}{X \text{ mL}}$

$100X = 75$

$\frac{100X}{100} = \frac{75}{100}$

$X = 0.75 \text{ mL}$

10. $1:3000 = \frac{1 \text{ g}}{3000 \text{ mL}} = \frac{1000 \text{ mg}}{3000 \text{ mL}} = \frac{1 \text{ mg}}{3 \text{ mL}}$

$\frac{1 \text{ mg}}{3 \text{ mL}} = \frac{0.5 \text{ mg}}{X \text{ mL}}$

$X = 1.5 \text{ mL}$

11. $20\% = \frac{20 \text{ g}}{100 \text{ mL}} = \frac{20,000 \text{ mg}}{100 \text{ mL}} = \frac{200 \text{ mg}}{1 \text{ mL}}$

$\frac{200 \text{ mg}}{1 \text{ mL}} = \frac{50 \text{ mg}}{X \text{ mL}}$

$200X = 50$

$\frac{200X}{200} = \frac{50}{200}$

$X = 0.25 \text{ mL or } 0.25 \text{ cc}$

12. $50\% = \frac{50 \text{ g}}{100 \text{ mL}} = \frac{1 \text{ g}}{2 \text{ mL}}$

$\frac{1 \text{ g}}{2 \text{ mL}} = \frac{2 \text{ g}}{X \text{ mL}}$

$X = 4 \text{ mL or } 4 \text{ cc}$

13. **70-30 insulin concentration means there is 70% NPH insulin and 30% Regular insulin in each unit.**

14. **10 units of Regular insulin and 20 units of NPH insulin in same syringe.**

a. **Draw back 20 units of air and insert into the NPH insulin vial (cloudy liquid).**

b. **Remove needle.**

   Draw back 10 units of air and inject into the Regular insulin vial (clear liquid) and leave needle in vial.

c. **Turn the vial of Regular insulin upside down and draw out 10 units of Regular insulin. Make sure all air bubbles are removed.**

d. **Roll the vial of NPH insulin in your hands to mix.**

e. **Insert needle into NPH vial and draw back to the 30 unit mark, since 10 units Regular + 20 units NPH = 30 units total.**

Chapter 9   Using the Formula Method to Calculate Dosages

1. $\dfrac{D}{H} \times Q = X$

   $\dfrac{\cancel{500} \text{ mg}}{\cancel{200} \text{ mg}} \times 1 \text{ mL} = 2.5 \text{ mL}$

2. $\dfrac{20 \text{ mg}}{5 \text{ mg}} \times 1 \text{ tab} = 4 \text{ tablets}$

3. $0.4 \text{ g} = 0.4 \times 1000 = 400 \text{ mg}$

   $\dfrac{400 \text{ mg}}{\underset{5}{\cancel{250} \text{ mg}}} \times \overset{1}{\cancel{5}} \text{ mL} = 8 \text{ mL}$

4. $\dfrac{\overset{3}{\cancel{15} \text{ mg}}}{\underset{4}{\cancel{20} \text{ mg}}} \times 1 \text{ mL} = 0.75 \text{ mL}$

5. $\dfrac{\overset{2}{\cancel{10} \text{ mg}}}{\underset{3}{\cancel{15} \text{ mg}}} \times 1 \text{ cc} = 0.67 \text{ cc}$

6. $\dfrac{60 \text{ mEq}}{\underset{8}{\cancel{80} \text{ mEq}}} \times \overset{1}{\cancel{10}} \text{ mL} = 7.5 \text{ mL}$

7. $\dfrac{0.25 \text{ mg}}{0.1 \text{ mg}} \times 1 \text{ mL} = 2.5 \text{ mL}$

8. $\dfrac{40 \text{ mg}}{10 \text{ mg}} \times 1 \text{ mL} = 4 \text{ mL}$

9. $\dfrac{500 \text{ mg}}{250 \text{ mg}} \times 1 \text{ tab} = 2 \text{ tablets}$

10. $\dfrac{3 \text{ mEq}}{0.45 \text{ mEq}} \times 1 \text{ mL} = 6.7 \text{ mL}$

Chapter 10   Pediatric Dosages

1. a. per day:

   Minimum per day: $\dfrac{20 \text{ mg}}{1 \text{ kg}} = \dfrac{X \text{ mg}}{10 \text{ kg}}$

   $X = 200 \text{ mg}$

   Maximum per day: $\dfrac{40 \text{ mg}}{1 \text{ kg}} = \dfrac{X \text{ mg}}{10 \text{ kg}}$

   $X = 400 \text{ mg}$

   Order is

   $100 \text{ mg q.8h} = \dfrac{100 \text{ mg}}{\text{dose}} \times \dfrac{3 \text{ doses}}{\text{day}} = 300 \text{ mg/day}$

   Dosage is within the recommended range.

   b. $\dfrac{125 \text{ mg}}{5 \text{ mL}} = \dfrac{100 \text{ mg}}{X \text{ mL}}$

   $125X = 500$

   $\dfrac{125X}{125} = \dfrac{500}{125}$

   $X = 4 \text{ mL}$

2. **Convert weight to kilograms:**

   $48 \text{ lb} = \dfrac{48}{2.2} = 21.8 = 22 \text{ kg}$

   Dosage to be administered:

   $\dfrac{3 \text{ mg}}{1 \text{ kg}} = \dfrac{X \text{ mg}}{22 \text{ kg}}$

   $X = 66 \text{ mg}$

   Amount to give:

   $\dfrac{80 \text{ mg}}{15 \text{ mL}} = \dfrac{66 \text{ mg}}{X \text{ mL}}$

   $80X = 990$

   $\dfrac{80X}{80} = \dfrac{990}{80}$

   $X = 12.4 \text{ mL}$

3. $\dfrac{80 \text{ mg}}{0.8 \text{ mL}} = \dfrac{30 \text{ mg}}{X}$

   $X = 0.3 \text{ mL}$

   Minimum: per dose $\dfrac{10 \text{ mg}}{1 \text{ kg}} = \dfrac{X \text{ mg}}{3 \text{ kg}}$

   $X = 30 \text{ mg}$

   Maximum: per dose $\dfrac{15 \text{ mg}}{1 \text{ kg}} = \dfrac{X \text{ mg}}{3 \text{ kg}}$

   $X = 45 \text{ mg}$

   Yes, the ordered amount of 30 mg for this child is safe.

4. **60 mg/m² × 0.6 m² = 36 mg**

5. **The child's BSA is 1.1 m²**
   250 mg/m² × 1.1 m² = 275 mg (child's dose)

6. **Convert 1 g to milligrams. 1 g = 1000 mg**
   $$\frac{0.27 \text{ m}^2}{1.7 \text{ m}^2} \times 1000 \text{ mg} = 158.8 \text{ or } 159 \text{ mg}$$

7. a. $\frac{0.38 \text{ m}^2}{1.7 \text{ m}^2} \times 250 \text{ mg} = 55.8 \text{ or } 56 \text{ mg}$

   b. $\frac{250 \text{ mg}}{5 \text{ mL}} = \frac{56 \text{ mg}}{X}$
      $$X = 1.1 \text{ mL}$$

8. a. **Determine BSA – 0.9 m².**
   $$\frac{0.90 \text{ m}^2}{1.7 \text{ m}^2} \times 0.25 \text{ mg} = 0.13 \text{ mg}$$
   (child's dosage)

   b. $\frac{0.25 \text{ mg}}{1 \text{ mL}} = \frac{0.13 \text{ mg}}{X \text{ mL}}$
      $$0.25X = 0.13$$
      $$\frac{0.25X}{0.25} = \frac{0.13}{0.25}$$
      $$X = 0.52 \text{ mL}$$

9. a. **Convert g to kg 1000 g = 1 kg**
      4000 g = 4 kg

      Minimum per day : $\frac{50 \text{ mg}}{1 \text{ kg}} = \frac{X \text{ mg}}{4 \text{ kg}}$
      $$X = 200 \text{ mg}$$

      Maximum per day : $\frac{100 \text{ mg}}{1 \text{ kg}} = \frac{X \text{ mg}}{4 \text{ kg}}$
      $$X = 400 \text{ mg}$$

   Infant should receive 200 mg–400 mg daily.
   Yes, the dosage is safe.

   b. **Convert 1 g to mg. 1 g = 1000 mg**
      One dose = 125 mg
      $$\frac{1000 \text{ mg}}{4 \text{ mL}} = \frac{125 \text{ mg}}{X \text{ mL}}$$
      $$1000X = 500$$
      $$\frac{1000X}{1000} = \frac{500}{1000}$$
      $$X = 0.5 \text{ mL}$$

10. a. **Convert 45 lb to kg**
       Equivalent 1 kg = 2.2 lb
       $$45 \text{ lb} = \frac{45}{2.2} = 20.4 \text{ or } 20 \text{ kg}$$

    Dosage range:

    Minimum per day : $\frac{6 \text{ mg}}{1 \text{ kg}} = \frac{X \text{ mg}}{20 \text{ kg}}$
    $$X = 120 \text{ mg}$$

    Minimum per dose : $\frac{120 \text{ mg}}{3 \text{ doses}} = 40 \text{ mg/dose}$

    Maximum per day : $\frac{7.5 \text{ mg}}{1 \text{ kg}} = \frac{X \text{ mg}}{20 \text{ kg}}$
    $$X = 150 \text{ mg}$$

    Maximum per dose : $\frac{150 \text{ mg}}{3 \text{ doses}} = 50 \text{ mg/dose}$

    Yes, the dosage is safe.

    b. **40 mg/mL since 10 mg/mL would require 2 injections.**

    c. $\frac{40 \text{ mg}}{1 \text{ mL}} = \frac{45 \text{ mg}}{X \text{ mL}}$
       $$40X = 45$$
       $$\frac{40X}{40} = \frac{45}{40}$$
       $$X = 1.1 \text{ mL}$$

11. **per day :** $\frac{30 \text{ mg}}{1 \text{ kg}} = \frac{X \text{ mg}}{12 \text{ kg}}$
    $$X = 360 \text{ mg}$$

    per dose : $\frac{360 \text{ mg}}{3 \text{ doses}} = 120 \text{ mg/dose}$

12. a. **Minimum per day :** $\frac{6 \text{ mg}}{1 \text{ kg}} = \frac{X \text{ mg}}{18 \text{ kg}}$
       $$X = 108 \text{ mg}$$

       Maximum per day : $\frac{12 \text{ mg}}{1 \text{ kg}} = \frac{X \text{ mg}}{18 \text{ kg}}$
       $$X = 216 \text{ mg}$$

    The child weighing 18 kg could receive 108–216 mg TMP daily.

    b. **Minimum per dose :** $\frac{108 \text{ mg}}{2 \text{ doses}} = 54 \text{ mg/dose}$

       Maximum per dose : $\frac{216 \text{ mg}}{2 \text{ doses}} = 108 \text{ mg/dose}$

    The child weighing 18 kg could receive 54–108 mg q.12 h

    c. $\frac{16 \text{ mg}}{1 \text{ mL}} = \frac{X \text{ mg}}{6 \text{ mL}}$
       $$X = 96 \text{ mg, yes the dosage is safe}$$

Chapter 11   Intravenous Calculations

1. **Convert 2 L to cc 1 L = 1000 cc**

$$\frac{2000 \text{ mL}}{24 \text{ h}} = 83.3 = 83 \text{ mL/h}$$

2. $$\frac{100 \text{ cc}}{45 \text{ minutes}} = \frac{X \text{ mL}}{60 \text{ min}}$$

$$\frac{45X}{45} = \frac{6000}{45}$$

$$45X = 6000$$

$$X = 133.3 \text{ or } 133$$

   Rate is 133 mL/h

3. $$\frac{1600 \text{ mL}}{18 \text{ h}} = 88.8 = 89$$

   Rate is 89 mL/h

4. **Time in minutes = 8 × 60 = 480 min**

$$\frac{V}{T} \times C = R$$

$$\frac{500 \text{ mL}}{480 \text{ min}} \times \frac{20 \text{ gtt}}{\text{mL}} = R$$

$$\frac{10,000}{480} = R$$

$$R = 20.8 \text{ or } 21 \text{ gtt/min}$$

5. **Time in minutes = 10 × 60 = 600 min**

$$\frac{1000 \text{ mL}}{600 \text{ min}} \times \frac{15 \text{ gtt}}{1 \text{ mL}} = R$$

$$\frac{150}{6} = R$$

$$R = 25 \text{ gtt/min}$$

6. **Constant: 6**

$$\frac{650 \text{ mL}}{4 \text{ h}} = 162.5 \text{ or } 163 \text{ mL/h}$$

$$\frac{\text{mL/h}}{\text{drop factor constant}} = \frac{\text{gtt}}{\text{min}}$$

$$\frac{163}{6} = 27 \text{ gtt/min}$$

7. **Constant: 4**

$$\frac{1000 \text{ mL}}{6 \text{ h}} = 166.6 \text{ or } 167 \text{ mL/h}$$

$$\frac{167}{4} = 41.7 \text{ or } 42 \text{ gtt/min}$$

8. **Constant: 1**

$$\frac{850 \text{ mL}}{8 \text{ h}} = 106.25 \text{ or } 106 \text{ mL/h}$$

$$\frac{106}{1} = 106 \text{ gtt/min}$$

9. **17 h = 1020 min**

$$\frac{V}{T} \times C = R$$

$$\frac{2500 \text{ mL}}{1020 \text{ min}} \times \frac{15 \text{ gtt}}{\text{mL}} = R$$

$$\frac{37500}{1020} = R$$

$$R = 36.7 \text{ or } \frac{37 \text{ gtt}}{\text{min}}$$

$$\frac{37 - 31}{31} = \frac{6}{31} = 0.19 = 19\%$$

   The rate needs to be increased to 37 gtt/min which is a 19% increase. This is within 25%, if allowable for the patient's condition and hospital policy.

10. $$\frac{V}{T} \times C = R$$

$$\frac{100 \text{ mL}}{60 \text{ min}} \times 20 \text{ gtt/mL} = R$$

$$R = \frac{2000}{60} = 33.3 \text{ or } 33 \text{ gtt/min}$$

11. $$\frac{V}{T} \times C = R$$

$$\frac{50 \text{ mL}}{40 \text{ min}} \times 10 \text{ gtt/mL} = R$$

$$\frac{500}{40} = R$$

$$R = 12.5 \text{ or } 13 \text{ gtt/min}$$

12. a. $$\frac{V}{T} \times C = R$$

$$\frac{50 \text{ mL}}{20 \text{ min}} \times 15 \text{ gtt/mL} = R$$

$$R = \frac{750}{20} = 37.5 \text{ or } 38 \text{ gtt/min}$$

   b. $$\frac{50 \text{ cc}}{20 \text{ min}} = \frac{X \text{ cc}}{60 \text{ min}}$$

$$20X = 3000$$

$$\frac{20X}{20} = \frac{3000}{20}$$

$$X = 150$$

   Rate = 150 mL/h

13. **Calculate the amount of dextrose and sodium chloride in 250 mL of D$_5$NS**

D$_5$ = Dextrose 5% = 5 g dextrose per 100 mL

$$\frac{5\text{ g}}{100\text{ mL}} = \frac{X\text{ g}}{250\text{ mL}}$$

$$100X = 1250$$

$$\frac{100X}{100} = \frac{1250}{100}$$

$$X = 12.5\text{ g dextrose}$$

NS = Normal Saline = 0.9%
$$= 0.9\text{ g NaCl per 100 mL}$$

$$\frac{0.9\text{ g}}{100\text{ mL}} = \frac{X\text{ g}}{250\text{ mL}}$$

$$100X = 225$$

$$\frac{100X}{100} = \frac{225}{100}$$

$$X = 2.25\text{ g NaCl}$$

Chapter 12   Advanced Intravenous Calculations

1. a. **100 mL + 20 mL = 120 mL**

 b.
$$\frac{V}{T} \times C = R$$

$$\frac{120\text{ mL}}{60\text{ min}} \times 60\text{ gtt/mL} = 120\text{ gtt/min}$$

 c.
$$\frac{1.5\text{ g}}{5\text{ mL}} = \frac{3\text{ g}}{X\text{ mL}}$$

$$1.5X = 15$$

$$\frac{1.5X}{1.5} = \frac{15}{1.5}$$

$$X = 10\text{ mL}$$

 d. **100 − 10 = 90 mL of NS**

2. a. **50 cc + 15 cc = 65 cc**

 b. $\frac{65\text{ mL}}{60\text{ min}} \times 60\text{ gtt/mL} = 65\text{ gtt/min}$

 c. **Equivalent: 1 g = 1000 mg**

 d.
$$\frac{1000\text{ mg}}{3\text{ cc}} = \frac{150\text{ mg}}{X\text{ cc}}$$

$$1000X = 450$$

$$\frac{1000X}{1000} = \frac{450}{1000}$$

$$X = 0.45\text{ cc}$$

 e. **50 − 0.45 = 49.55 cc**

3. a.
$$\frac{40\text{ mEq}}{1000\text{ cc}} = \frac{X\text{ mEq}}{500\text{ cc}}$$

$$1000X = 20000$$

$$\frac{1000X}{1000} = \frac{20,000}{1000}$$

$$X = 20\text{ mEq KCl}$$

 b.
$$\frac{80\text{ mEq}}{10\text{ cc}} = \frac{20\text{ mEq}}{X\text{ cc}}$$

$$80X = 200$$

$$\frac{80X}{80} = \frac{200}{80}$$

$$X = 2.5\text{ cc}$$

 c.
$$\frac{20\text{ mEq}}{500\text{ mL}} = \frac{X\text{ mEq}}{25\text{ mL}}$$

$$500X = 500$$

$$\frac{500X}{500} = \frac{500}{500}$$

$$X = 1\text{ mEq}$$

 Patient will receive 1 mEq/h.

4.
$$\frac{20,000\text{ U}}{250\text{ mL}} = \frac{500\text{ U/h}}{X\text{ mL/h}}$$

$$20,000X = 125,000$$

$$\frac{20,000X}{20,000} = \frac{125,000}{20,000}$$

$$X = 6.25\text{ or } 6\text{ mL/h}$$

 The drop factor is 20 gtt/mL.

$$\frac{6\text{ mL}}{60\text{ min}} \times 20\text{ gtt/mL} = 2\text{ gtt/min}$$

5.
$$\frac{30000\text{ U}}{500\text{ cc}} = \frac{X\text{ U/h}}{10\text{ cc/h}}$$

$$500X = 300,000$$

$$\frac{500X}{500} = \frac{300,000}{500}$$

$$X = 600\text{ U per hour}$$

6.
$$\frac{100\text{ mg}}{50\text{ cc}} = \frac{4\text{ mg/h}}{X\text{ cc/h}}$$

$$100X = 200$$

$$\frac{100X}{100} = \frac{200}{100}$$

$$X = 2\text{ cc per hour}$$

7.
$$\frac{65\text{ cc}}{1\text{ h}} = \frac{2000\text{ cc}}{X\text{ h}}$$

$$65X = 2000$$

$$\frac{65X}{65} = \frac{2000}{65}$$

$$X = 30.8\text{ hours or } 30\text{ hours } 48\text{ minutes}$$

8. $\dfrac{150 \text{ mL}}{T} \times 15 \text{ gtt/mL} = 30 \text{ gtt/min}$

$$\dfrac{2250}{T} = \dfrac{30}{1}$$

$$30T = 2250$$

$$\dfrac{30T}{30} = \dfrac{2250}{30}$$

$$T = 75 \text{ minutes}$$

9. $\dfrac{V \text{ mL}}{720 \text{ min}} \times \dfrac{10 \text{ gtt}}{1 \text{ mL}} = 40 \text{ gtt/min}$

$$\dfrac{10V}{720} = \dfrac{40}{1}$$

$$10V = 28800$$

$$\dfrac{10V}{10} = \dfrac{28800}{10}$$

$$V = 2880 \text{ mL in 12 hours}$$

10. $\dfrac{23 \text{ mg}}{1 \text{ min}} = \dfrac{X \text{ mg}}{60 \text{ min}}$

$$X = 1380 \text{ mg}$$

Patient must receive 1380 mg/h.

Determine mL/h.

Convert 1 g to mg. Equivalent: 1 g = 1000 mg.

$$\dfrac{1000 \text{ mg}}{100 \text{ mL}} = \dfrac{1380 \text{ mg}}{X \text{ mL}}$$

$$1000X = 138000$$

$$\dfrac{1000X}{1000} = \dfrac{138000}{1000}$$

$$X = 138 \text{ mL}$$

Rate must be 138 mL/h.

11. a. $75 \text{ lb} = \dfrac{75}{2.2} = 34 \text{ kg}$

$$\dfrac{0.1 \text{ U}}{1 \text{ kg}} = \dfrac{X \text{ U}}{34 \text{ kg}}$$

$$X = 3.4 \text{ U}$$

3.4 U must be infused per minute.

b. $\dfrac{3.4 \text{ U}}{1 \text{ min}} = \dfrac{X \text{ U}}{60 \text{ min}}$

$$X = 204 \text{ U}$$

204 U must be infused per hour.

c. $\dfrac{50 \text{ U}}{100 \text{ mL}} = \dfrac{204 \text{ U}}{X \text{ mL}}$

$$50X = 20400$$

$$\dfrac{50X}{50} = \dfrac{20400}{50}$$

$$X = 408 \text{ mL}$$

Rate is 408 mL/h

12. a. $\dfrac{50 \text{ mL}}{\overset{}{\underset{4}{\cancel{60} \text{ min}}}} \times \dfrac{\overset{1}{\cancel{15} \text{ gtt}}}{\text{min}} = 12.5 \text{ or } 13 \text{ gtt/min}$

b. **Gentamycin 40 mg 2 times/24 h = Gentamycin 40 mg to run 2 h/24 h**

c. **$2 \times 50 = 100 \text{ cc}$**

d. **$1500 - 100 = 1400 \text{ cc}$**

e. **$24 - 2 = 22 \text{ h}$**

f. $\dfrac{1400 \text{ cc}}{1320 \text{ min}} \times 15 \text{ gtt/min} = \dfrac{21000}{3120} = 15.9 \text{ or } 16 \text{ gtt/min}$

g. **IV PB rate = 13 gtt/min**

13. $\dfrac{40 \text{ mg}}{1 \text{ mL}} = \dfrac{30 \text{ mg}}{X \text{ mL}}$

$$\dfrac{40X}{40} = \dfrac{30}{40}$$

$$40X = 30$$

$$X = 0.75 \text{ or } 0.8 \text{ mL}$$

14. For the first 10 kg,

$$\dfrac{100 \text{ mL}}{1 \text{ kg}} = \dfrac{X \text{ mL}}{10 \text{ kg}}$$

$$X = 1000 \text{ mL}$$

For the next 10 kg,

$$\dfrac{50 \text{ mL}}{1 \text{ kg}} = \dfrac{X \text{ mL}}{10 \text{ kg}}$$

$$X = 500 \text{ mL}$$

For the last 2 kg,

$$\dfrac{20 \text{ mL}}{1 \text{ kg}} = \dfrac{X \text{ mL}}{2 \text{ kg}}$$

$$X = 40 \text{ mL}$$

per day,

$$1000 \text{ mL} + 500 \text{ mL} + 40 \text{ mL} = 1540 \text{ mL}$$

$$\dfrac{1540 \text{ mL}}{24 \text{ h}} = \dfrac{X \text{ mL}}{1 \text{ h}}$$

$$24X = 1540$$

$$\dfrac{24X}{24} = \dfrac{1540}{24}$$

$$X = 64.2$$

$$\text{Rate} = 64 \text{ mL/h}$$

Part 4   Transparency Masters

Converting and Reducing Fractions

■ **To convert a mixed number to an improper fraction, multiply the whole number by the denominator and add the numerator.**

Example: $1\frac{1}{3} = \frac{4}{3}$

■ **To convert an improper fraction to a mixed number, divide the numerator by the denominator.**

Example: $\frac{20}{9} = 2\frac{2}{9}$

■ **To reduce a fraction to lowest terms, divide both terms by the largest whole number that will divide evenly. Value remains the same.**

Example: $\frac{6}{10} = \frac{3}{5}$

■ **To enlarge a fraction, multiply both terms by the same number. Value remains the same.**

Example: $\frac{1}{12} = \frac{2}{24}$

Fractions and Mathematical Operations

- *To add or subtract fractions,* convert to equivalent fractions with like denominators, then add or subtract the numerators.

- *To multiply fractions,* multiply numerators and multiply denominators.

- *To divide fractions,* invert the divisor and multiply.

- Reduce results to lowest terms.

Decimals and Mathematical Operations

■ To multiply decimals, place the decimal point in the product to the *left* as many decimal places as there are in the two decimals multiplied.

Example: $0.25 \times 0.2 = 0.050 = 0.05$

■ To divide decimals, move the decimal point in the divisor and dividend the number of decimal places that will make the divisor a whole number.

Example: $1.2,\overline{)24.0.}$ with quotient $20.$

■ To multiply or divide decimals by powers of 10, move the decimal to the *right* (to *multiply*) or to the *left* (to *divide*) the number of decimal places as there are zeros in the multiple of 10.

Examples: $5.06 \times 10 = 5.0.6 = 50.6$;

$2.1 \div 100 = .02.1 = 0.021$

■ When rounding decimals, add 1 to the place value considered if the next decimal place is 5 or greater.

Examples:
(rounded to hundredths) $3.054 = 3.05$; $0.566 = 0.57$;
(rounded to tenths) $3.05 = 3.1$; $0.54 = 0.5$

Decimal and Percent Conversions

■ **To change a percent to a decimal fraction, move the decimal point two places to the left.**

Example: $4\% = .04. = 0.04$

■ **To change a decimal fraction to a percent, move the decimal point two places to the right.**

Example: $0.04 = 0.04. = 4\%$

Rules of Metric Notation

1. **The unit or abbreviation always follows the amount.**

    Example: 5 g, NOT g 5.

2. **Decimals are used to designate fractional metric units.**

    Example: 1.5 mL, not $1\frac{1}{2}$ mL.

3. **Use a zero to emphasize the decimal point for fractional metric units of less than 1.**

    Example: 0.5 mg, NOT .5 mg.

    This is a critical rule as it will prevent confusion and potential dosage error. Consider for a moment if you overlooked the decimal point and misinterpreted the medication order as 5 mg instead of 0.5 mg. The patient would be overdosed 10 times.

4. **Omit unnecessary zeros.**

    Example: 1.5 g, NOT 1.50 g.

    This is another critical rule.

5. **When in doubt, double check, and ask the writer for clarification.**

Metric Units of Measurement and Equivalents

Unit	Abbreviation	Equivalents
Weight		
gram	g	1 g = 1000 mg
milligram	mg	1 mg = 1000 mcg, or 0.001 g
microgram	mcg (mg)	1 mcg = 0.001 mg = 0.000001 g
kilogram	kg	1 kg = 1000 g
Volume		
liter	L (or ℓ)	1 L = 1000 mL
milliliter	mL (or mℓ)	1 mL = 0.001 L or 1 cc
cubic centimeter	cc	1 cc = 1 mL or 0.001 L
Length		
meter	m	1 m = 100 cm, or 1000 mm
centimeter	cm	1 cm = 0.01 m, or 10 mm
millimeter	mm	1 mm = 0.001 m, or 0.1 cm

Metric System Review

In the metric system:

- The metric base units are gram, liter, and meter.

- Subunits are designated by the appropriate prefix and the base unit, such as *milli*gram.

- The unit or abbreviation always follows the amount.

- Decimals are used to designate fractional amounts.

- Use a zero to emphasize the decimal point for fractional amounts of less than 1.

- Omit unnecessary zeros.

- Multiply or divide by 1000 to derive most equivalents needed for dosage calculations. 1 cc = 1 mL.

- When in doubt about the exact amount or the abbreviation used, do not guess. Ask the writer to clarify.

Apothecary System of Measurement

In the apothecary system:

- ■ The common units for dosage calculations are grain and ounce.

- ■ The quantity is best expressed in lowercase Roman numerals. Amounts greater than ten may be expressed in Arabic numbers, *except* 20 (xx) and 30 (xxx).

- ■ Quantities of less than one are expressed as fractions, *except* $\frac{1}{2}$.

- ■ One-half ($\frac{1}{2}$) is expressed by the symbol *ss*.

- ■ The abbreviation or symbol is clearly written before the quantity.

- ■ If you are unsure about the exact meaning of any medical notation, do not guess or assume; ask the writer for clarification.

Apothecary and Household Systems of Measurement

APOTHECARY

Unit	Abbreviation	Equivalents
quarter	qt	qt i = pt ii
pint	pt	qt i = ℥ 32
fluid ounce	℥	pt i = ℥ 16
dram	ʒ	
minim	♏	

HOUSEHOLD

Unit	Abbreviation	Equivalent
drop	gtt	
teaspoon	tsp (or t)	1 T = 3 t
tablespoon	tbs (or T)	

Converting Within the Metric System Using Ratio and Proportion

To convert between metric units:

■ **Recall the metric equivalents.**

■ **Follow the rule: Ratio for known equivalent equals ratio for unknown equivalent.**

■ **Label the units and match the units in the numerators and denominators.**

■ **Cross-multiply to find the value of the unknown X.**

Approximate Equivalents

1 g = gr 15   1 L = qt i = pt ii = ℥ 32 = 4 cups

gr i = 60 mg   pt i = 500 mL = ℥ 16 = 2 cups

1 t = 5 mL   1 cup = 250 mL = ℥ viii

1 T = 3 t = 15 mL = ℥ ss   1 kg = 2.2 lb

℥ i = 30 mL = 6 t   1 in = 2.5 cm

Weight and Volume Equivalents

WEIGHT EQUIVALENTS

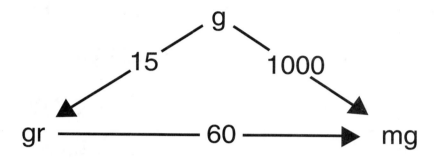

VOLUME EQUIVALENTS

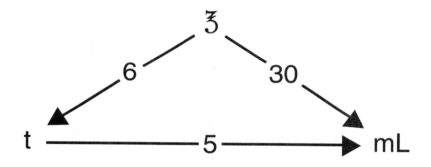

Using Ratio and Proportion to Convert between Systems of Measurement

To use the ratio and proportion method to convert between systems of measurement:

■ Recall the approximate equivalents.

■ Follow the rule: Ratio for known equivalent equals ratio for unknown equivalent.

■ Label and match units in the numerators and denominators.

■ Cross-multiply to solve for the unknown X.

Comparison of Traditional and 24-Hour Time

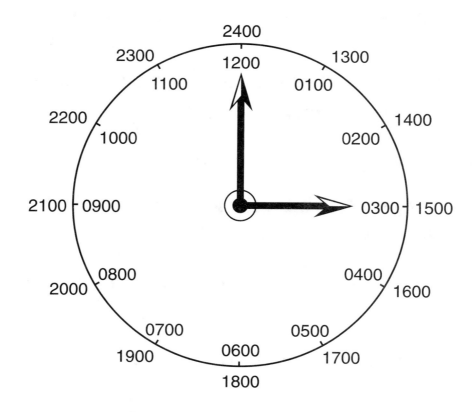

AM	Int'l. Time	PM	Int'l. Time
12 midnight	2400	12 Noon	1200
1	0100	1	1300
2	0200	2	1400
3	0300	3	1500
4	0400	4	1600
5	0500	5	1700
6	0600	6	1800
7	0700	7	1900
8	0800	8	2000
9	0900	9	2100
10	1000	10	2200
11	1100	11	2300

Converting between Celsius and Fahrenheit Temperature Scales

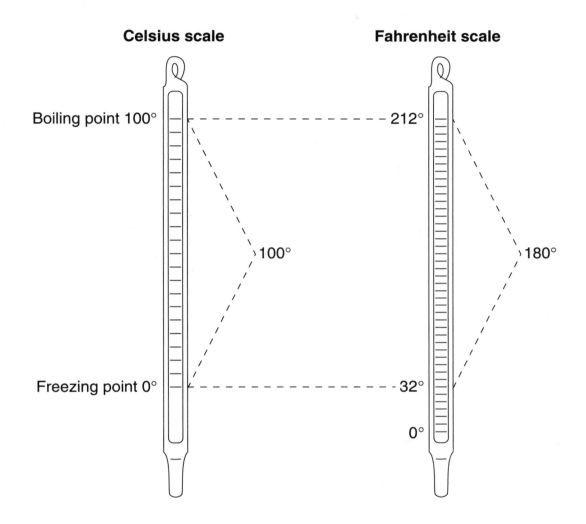

Use these formulas to convert between Fahrenheit and Celsius temperatures:

■ $°C = \dfrac{°F - 32}{1.8}$

■ $°F = 1.8°C + 32$

Medicine Cups

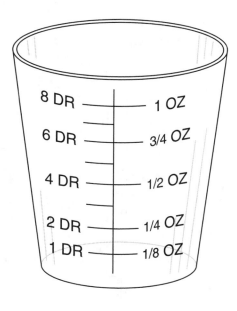

8 DR — 1 OZ
6 DR — 3/4 OZ
4 DR — 1/2 OZ
2 DR — 1/4 OZ
1 DR — 1/8 OZ

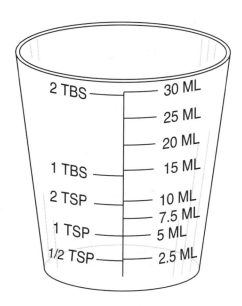

2 TBS — 30 ML
— 25 ML
— 20 ML
1 TBS — 15 ML
2 TSP — 10 ML
— 7.5 ML
1 TSP — 5 ML
1/2 TSP — 2.5 ML

Equipment Used in Dosage Measurement

■ The medicine cup has a 1-ounce or 30-milliliter capacity for oral liquids. It is also calibrated to measure teaspoons, tablespoons, and drams. Amounts less than 2.5 milliliters should be measured in a smaller device, such as an oral syringe.

■ The calibrated dropper measures small amounts of oral liquids. The size of the drop varies according to the diameter of the dropper.

■ The standard 3-cc syringe is used to measure most injectable drugs. It is calibrated in tenths of a cc.

■ The prefilled, single-dose syringe is to be used once and discarded.

■ The standard U-100 insulin syringe is used to measure U-100 insulin only. It is calibrated for a total of 100 units or 1 cc.

■ The Lo-Dose® U-100 insulin syringe is used for measuring small amounts of U-100 insulin. It is calibrated for a total of 50 units or 0.5 cc. A smaller Lo-Dose® U-100 insulin syringe is calibrated for 30 units or 0.3 cc. This syringe is commonly used for administering insulin to children.

■ The tuberculin syringe is used to measure small or critical amounts of injectable drugs. It is calibrated in hundredths of a mL for a total of 0.5 mL or 1 mL.

■ Do not use syringes intended for injections in the administration of oral medications.

3 cc, 5 cc, 10 cc, and 20 cc Syringes

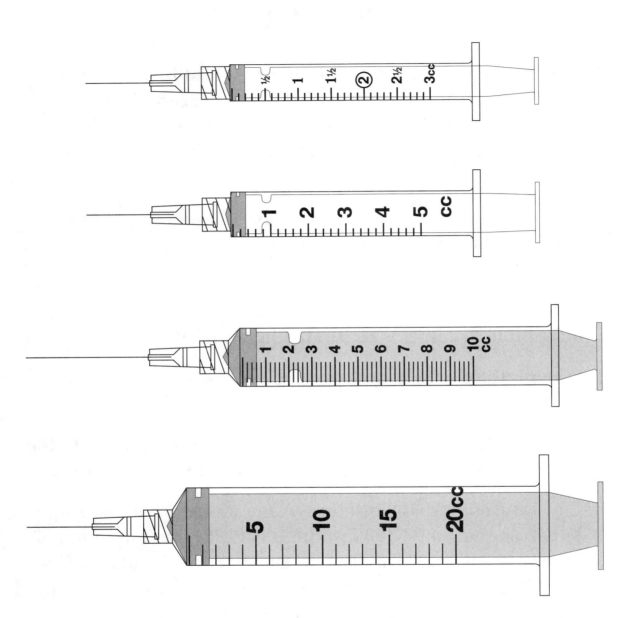

0.5 mL and 1.0 mL Tuberculin Syringes

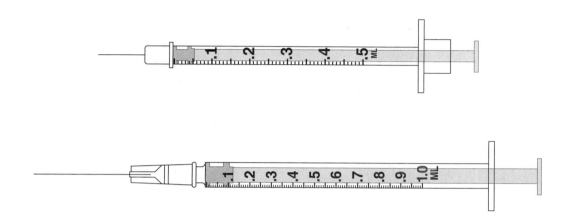

30 Unit, 50 Unit, and 100 Unit Insulin Syringes

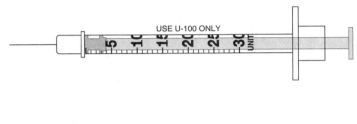

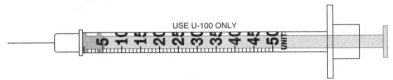

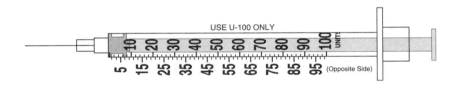

Sample Medication Labels

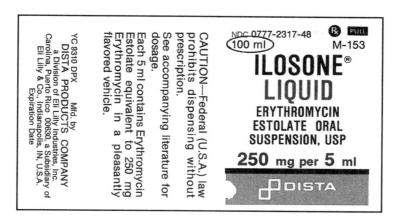

YC 9310-DPX
Mfd. by
DISTA PRODUCTS COMPANY
a Division of Eli Lilly Industries, Inc.
Carolina, Puerto Rico 00630, a Subsidiary of
Eli Lilly & Co., Indianapolis, IN, U.S.A.
Expiration Date

CAUTION—Federal (U.S.A.) law
prohibits dispensing without
prescription.
See accompanying literature for
dosage.
Each 5 ml contains Erythromycin
Estolate equivalent to 250 mg
Erythromycin in a pleasantly
flavored vehicle.

NDC 0777-2317-48
100 ml
M-153
Rx PULL

ILOSONE®
LIQUID
ERYTHROMYCIN
ESTOLATE ORAL
SUSPENSION, USP
250 mg per 5 ml
DISTA

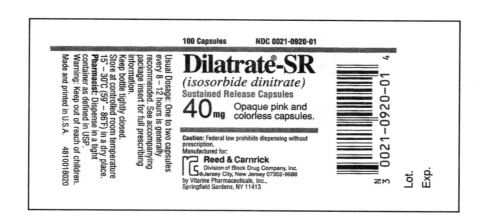

100 Capsules   NDC 0021-0920-01

Dilatrate®-SR
(isosorbide dinitrate)
Sustained Release Capsules
40 mg   Opaque pink and
colorless capsules.

Caution: Federal law prohibits dispensing without
prescription.
Manufactured for:
Reed & Carnrick
Division of Block Drug Company, Inc.
Jersey City, New Jersey 07302-9988
by Vitarine Pharmaceuticals, Inc.,
Springfield Gardens, NY 11413

Usual Dosage: One to two capsules
every 8 - 12 hours is generally
recommended. See accompanying
package insert for full prescribing
information.
Keep bottle tightly closed.
Store at controlled room temperature
15° – 30°C (59° – 86°F) in a dry place.
Pharmacist: Dispense in a tight
container as defined in USP.
Warning: Keep out of reach of children.
Made and printed in U.S.A.   4810018020

0021-0920-01 4
N 3
Lot.
Exp.

Sample Medication Labels

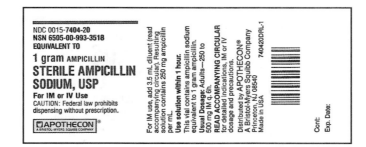

NDC 0015-7404-20
NSN 6505-00-993-3518
EQUIVALENT TO

1 gram AMPICILLIN

STERILE AMPICILLIN SODIUM, USP

For IM or IV Use
CAUTION: Federal law prohibits dispensing without prescription.

APOTHECON®
A BRISTOL-MYERS SQUIBB COMPANY

For IM use, add 3.5 mL diluent (read accompanying circular). Resulting solution contains 250 mg ampicillin per mL.
Use solution within 1 hour.
This vial contains ampicillin sodium equivalent to 1 gram ampicillin.
Usual Dosage: Adults—250 to 500 mg IM q. 6h.
READ ACCOMPANYING CIRCULAR for detailed indications, IM or IV dosage and precautions.
Distributed by APOTHECON®
A Bristol-Myers Squibb Company
Princeton, NJ 08540
Made in USA

74042ODRL-1

Cont:
Exp. Date:

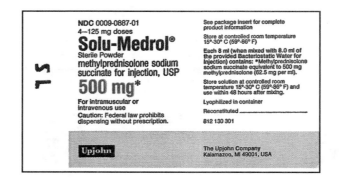

NDC 0009-0887-01
4—125 mg doses

Solu-Medrol®
Sterile Powder
methylprednisolone sodium succinate for injection, USP

500 mg*

For intramuscular or intravenous use
Caution: Federal law prohibits dispensing without prescription.

Upjohn

See package insert for complete product information

Store at controlled room temperature 15°-30° C (59°-86° F)

Each 8 ml (when mixed with 8.0 ml of the provided Bacteriostatic Water for Injection) contains: *Methylprednisolone sodium succinate equivalent to 500 mg methylprednisolone (62.5 mg per ml).

Store solution at controlled room temperature 15°-30° C (59°-86° F) and use within 48 hours after mixing.

Lyophilized in container
Reconstituted _____

812 130 301

The Upjohn Company
Kalamazoo, MI 49001, USA

Sample Medication Labels

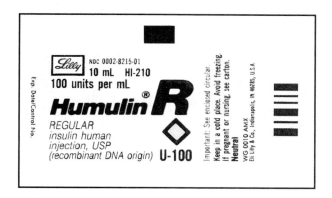

2 mL
LANOXIN®
(DIGOXIN)
INJECTION
500 µg (0.5 mg)
in 2 mL
(250 µg [0.25 mg] per mL)
DILUTION NOT REQUIRED
PROPYLENE GLYCOL 40%
ALCOHOL 10%
Store at 15° to 25°C (59° to
77°F). Protect from light.

FOR I.V. OR I.M. USE
BURROUGHS WELLCOME CO.
Research Triangle Park, NC 27709
542282

LOT
EXP.

Lilly NDC 0002-8215-01
10 mL HI-210
100 units per mL

Humulin R®

REGULAR
insulin human
injection, USP
(recombinant DNA origin) U-100

Neutral

Important: See enclosed circular.
Keep in a cold place. Avoid freezing.
If pregnant or nursing, see carton.

WG 0010 AMX
Eli Lilly & Co., Indianapolis, IN 46285, U.S.A.

Exp. Date/Control No.

Sample Medication Labels

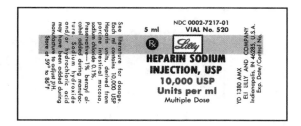

Label Review

Read labels carefully to:

■ identify the drug and the manufacturer.

■ differentiate between dosage strength, form, supply dosage, total container volume, and administration route.

■ find the directions for reconstitution, as needed.

■ note expiration date.

■ describe lot or control number.

Medication Administration Record (MAR)
(Noncomputer Version)

MEDICATION ADMINISTRATION RECORD

ORIGINAL ORDER DATE	DATE STARTED / RENEWED	MEDICATION - DOSAGE	ROUTE	SCHEDULE 11-7	7-3	3-11	DATE 11-3-xx 11-7	7-3	3-11	DATE 11-4-xx 11-7	7-3	3-11	DATE 11-5-xx 11-7	7-3	3-11	DATE 11-6-xx 11-7	7-3	3-11
11-3	11-3	Keflex 250 mg q. 6 h	PO	12 / 6	12	6		GP 12	MS 6	12JJ 6JJ	GP 12	MS 6						
11-3	11-4	Human NPH Insulin 40 U ā breakfast	SC		7³⁰						GP 7³⁰ Ⓡ							
11-3	11-3	Lasix 40 mg q.d.	PO		9			GP 9			GP 9							
11-3	11-3	Slow-K 8 mEq b.i.d.	PO		9	9			MS 9		GP 9	MS 9						
		PRN																
11-3	11-3	Demerol 75 mg q. 3-4 h	IM	severe pain				GP 12Ⓛ	MS 6Ⓜ-10 Ⓙ									
11-3	11-4	Codeine 30 mg q. 4 h	PO	mild-mod pain						JJ 6	GP 2							
11-3	11-3	Tylenol 650 mg q. 4 h	PO	fever >101°F				GP 12	MS 4-8	JJ 12-4	GP 8-12							

INJECTION SITES

B - RIGHT ARM	D - RIGHT ANTERIOR THIGH	H - LEFT ABDOMEN	L - LEFT BUTTOCKS
C - RIGHT ABDOMEN	G - LEFT ARM	J - LEFT ANTERIOR THIGH	M - RIGHT BUTTOCKS

DATE GIVEN	TIME	INT.	ONE - TIME MEDICATION - DOSAGE	RT.	SCHEDULE 11-7	7-3	3-11	DATE 11-7	7-3	3-11	DATE 11-7	7-3	3-11	DATE 11-7	7-3	3-11
11-3	2200ms		Lasix 80 mg stat	IV												

SIGNATURE OF NURSE ADMINISTERING MEDICATIONS

11-7		JJ J. Jones, LPN
7-3	GP G. Pickar, RN	GP G. Pickar, RN
3-11	MS M. Smith, RN	MS M. Smith, RN

DATE GIVEN	TIME	INT.	MEDICATION-DOSAGE-CONT.	RT.

RECOPIED BY:

CHECKED BY:

Patient, Mary Q.

#3-11316-7

ALLERGIES: None Known

(1) ORIGINAL COPY

602-31 (7-92) (MPC# 1355)

LITHO IN U.S.A. K6508 (7-92) D39553B

© 1999 Delmar Publishers, Albany, NY

Medication Administration Record (MAR)
(Computer Version)

PHARMACY MAR

START	STOP	MEDICATION	SCHEDULED TIMES	OK'D BY	0001 HRS. TO 1200 HRS.	1201 HRS. TO 2400 HRS.
08/31/xx 1800 SCH		PROCAN SR 500 MG TAB-SR 500 MG Q6H PO	0600 1200 1800 2400	JD	0600GP 1200 GP	1800 MS 2400 JD
09/03/xx 0900 SCH		DIGOXIN (LANOXIN) 0.125 MG TAB 1 TAB QOD PO ODD DAYS-SEPT	0900	JD	0900 GP	
09/03/xx 0900 SCH		FUROSEMIDE (LASIX) 40 MG TAB 1 TAB QD PO	0900	JD	0900 GP	
09/03/xx 0845 SCH		REGLAN 10 MG TAB 10 MG AC&HS PO GIVE ONE NOW!!	0730 1130 1630 2100	JD	0730 GP 1130 GP	1630 MS 2100 MS
09/04/xx 0900 SCH		K-LYTE 25 MEQ EFFERVESCENT TAB 1 EFF. TAB BID PO DISSOLVE AS DIR START 9-4	0900 1700	JD	0900 GP	1700 GP
09/03/xx 1507 PRN		NITROGLYCERIN 1/50 GR 0.4 MG TAB-SL 1 TABLET PRN* SL PRN CHEST PAIN		JD		
09/03/xx 1700 PRN		DARVOCET-N 100* 1 TAB Q4-6H PO PRN MILD–MODERATE PAIN		JD		
09/03/xx 2100 PRN		MEPERIDINE* (DEMEROL) INJ 50 MG Q4H IM PRN SEVERE PAIN W PHENERGAN		JD		2200 Ⓗ MS
09/03/xx 2100 PRN		PROMETHAZINE (PHENERGAN) INJ 50 MG Q4H IM PRN SEVERE PAIN W DEMEROL		JD		2200 Ⓗ MS

Gluteus	Thigh
A. Right	H. Right
B. Left	I. Left
Ventro Gluteal	
C. Right	J. Right
D. Left	K. Left
E. Abdomen 1|2	
3|4	

730-13 (12/83)

	NURSE'S SIGNATURE	INITIAL
7–3	G. Pickar, R.N.	GP
3–11	M. Smith, R.N.	MS
11–7	J. Doe, R.N.	JD

ALLERGIES: **NKA**

DIAGNOSIS: **CHF**

Patient: *Patient, John D.*
Patient #: 3-81512-3
Admitted: 08/31/xx
Physician: *J. Physician, MD*
Room: PCU-14 PCU

Examining Drug Orders

■ All parts of the drug order must be stated clearly, for accurate, exact interpretation. If you are ever in doubt as to the meaning or any part of a drug order, ask the writer to clarify.

Parts of the Drug Order

1. Name of the patient

2. Name of the drug to be administered

3. Dosage of the drug

4. Route by which the drug is to be administered

5. Time and/or frequency of administration

    — 5 Rights

6. Date and time when the order was written

7. Signature of the person writing the order

Items 1–5 = Rights of Safe Medication Administration

    1. RIGHT patient

    2. RIGHT drug

    3. RIGHT dosage

    4. RIGHT route

    5. RIGHT time/frequency

Three Steps to Dosage Calculation

To calculate the correct dosage of the medication ordered, use the following three simple steps.

Step 1. *Convert:* **Be sure that all measures are in the same system, and all units are in the same size, converting when necessary.**

Step 2. *Think:* **Carefully estimate what is a reasonable amount of the drug that should be administered.**

Step 3. *Calculate:* **Compute the drug dosage using the ratio for the drug you have on hand as equivalent to the ratio for the desired drug.**

Three Steps to Dosage Calculation

Step 1. *Convert:* to units of the same system and same size.

Step 2. *Think:* learn to reason for the logical answer.

Step 3. *Calculate:* $\dfrac{\text{Dosage on hand}}{\text{Amount on hand}} = \dfrac{\text{Dosage desired}}{\text{X Amount desired}}$

■ For most problems, convert to:

1. supply dosage you have on hand (gr → mg)

2. smaller size unit (g → mg)

Ratio for Drug on Hand =
Ratio for Drug Desired

Ratio for drug you have on hand equals ratio for the desired drug.

Look again at Steps 1 through 3 as a valuable dosage calculation checklist.

■ **Step 1.** *Convert:* **Be sure that all measures are in the same system, and all units are in the same size.**

■ **Step 2.** *Think:* **Carefully consider the reasonable amount of the drug that should be administered.**

■ **Step 3.** *Calculate:* $\dfrac{\text{Dosage on hand}}{\text{Amount on hand}} = \dfrac{\text{Dosage desired}}{\text{X Amount desired}}$

Calculating Drug Dosages

■ You cannot calculate drug dosages unless all
units of measure are in the same system and
the same size. Regardless of which method you
use (formula or ratio-proportion), the first step
is to always CONVERT, the second step is to
always THINK or reason for the logical answer
and the third step is to CALCULATE the
amount to give.

Reconstitution of Drugs

It is important that you remember the following points when reconstituting drugs:

■ If any medicine remains for future use after reconstitution, clearly label:
1. *strength* or concentration per volume
2. *date* and *time* of preparation
3. *initials* of individual performing procedure

■ Read all instructions carefully! If no instructions accompany the vial, confer with the pharmacist before proceeding.

■ Prepare a maximum of 3 mL per intramuscular injection site for an average size adult, 2 mL per site for children ages 6–12, and 1 mL for an infant to a 5 year old.

■ When calculating fractional dosages that will be measured in syringes, give answers in decimal form to the closest amount that can be measured by that syringe, such as 1.5 mL as measured in a 3-cc syringe or 0.25 cc as measured in a tuberculin syringe.

■ Round standard injection dosages over 1 mL to tenths and measure in the 3-cc syringe. The 3-cc syringe is calibrated in 0.1 cc increments.

■ Round small (less than 1 mL), critical care, or children's dosages to hundredths and measure in the tuberculin syringe. The tuberculin syringes are calibrated in 0.01 mL increments.

■ Measure amounts less than 0.5 mL in the tuberculin syringe.

Nomogram for Estimating Body Surface Area

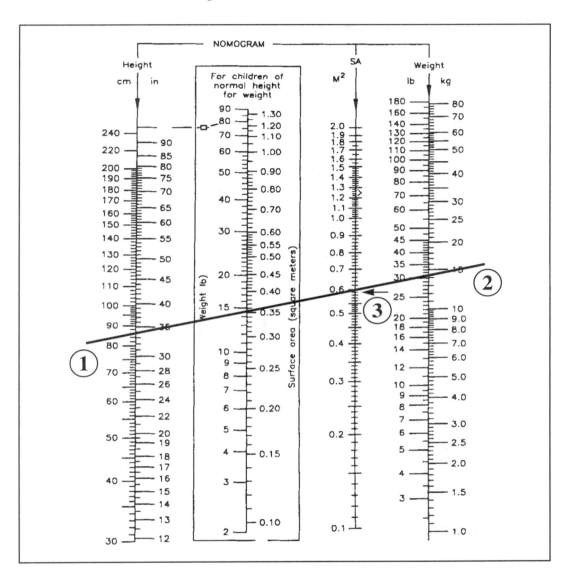

West's Nomogram for Estimation of Body Surface Area

Body surface area (BSA) is determined by drawing a straight line from the patient's height ① in the far left column to his or her weight ② in the far right column. Intersection of the line with the body surface area (BSA) column ③ is the estimated BSA (m²). For infants and children of normal height for weight, BSA may be estimated from weight alone by referring to the enclosed area.

(Reprinted with permission from Behrman, R. E. and Vaughan, V. C., Nelson Textbook of Pediatrics, 15th ed., 1996, W. B. Saunders Company, Philadelphia, PA 19105.)

Nomogram for Estimating Body Surface Area

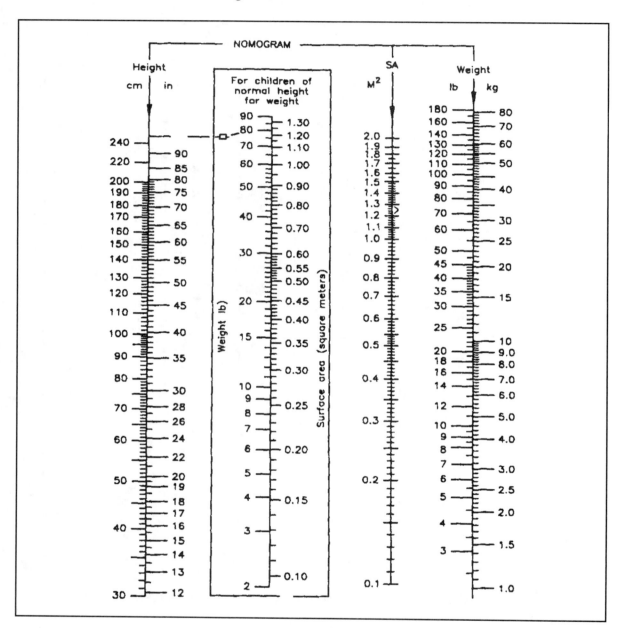

West's Nomogram for Estimation of Body Surface Area

(Reprinted with permission from Behrman, R. E. and Vaughan, V. C., Nelson Textbook of Pediatrics, *15th ed., 1996, W. B. Saunders Company, Philadelphia, PA 19105.)*

Regulating, Calculating, and Monitoring IV Flow Rate

■ **When regulating IV flow rate for an electronic infusion device, calculate mL/h.**

■ **When calculating IV flow rate to regulate an IV manually, find the drop factor and calculate gtt/min by using the:**

Formula Method

$$\frac{V}{T} \times C = R$$

or Short Cut Method

$$\frac{mL/h}{\text{Drop factor constant}} = gtt/min$$

■ **Carefully monitor patients receiving intravenous fluids at least hourly.**

■ **Check remaining IV fluids.**

■ **Check IV flow rate.**

■ **Observe IV site for complications.**

Recalculating Manually Regulated IVs

■ **For manually regulated IVs, recalculate flow rate when off schedule, if permitted by the hospital policy:**

$$\frac{\text{New flow rate} - \text{Ordered flow rate}}{\text{Ordered flow rate}} = \% \text{ Variation}$$

■ **Recalculated flow rate must not vary from the original rate by more than 25 percent if allowed by hospital policy. Do not arbitrarily speed up or slow down to catch up.**

Formulas for Calculating IV Infusion Time

■ **The formula to calculate IV infusion time, when mL/h is known:**

$$\frac{\text{TOTAL volume}}{\text{mL/h}} = \text{TOTAL hours}$$

■ **The formula to calculate IV infusion time, when flow rate (gtt/min) and drop factor (gtt/mL) are known:**

$$\frac{V}{T} \times C = R$$

"T" is the unknown.

■ **The formula to calculate IV volume, when flow rate (gtt/min), drop factor (gtt/mL), and time are known:**

$$\frac{V}{T} \times C = R$$

"V" is the unknown.

Rules for IV Calculations—
Infusion Devices

To regulate an IV by electronic infusion pump or controller, calibrated in mL/h,

$$\frac{\text{Total mL ordered}}{\text{Total h ordered}} = \text{mL/h (rounded to a whole number)}$$

Rules for IV Calculations— Flow Rate

The formula for IV flow rate is:

$$\frac{V}{T} \times C = R$$

In this formula:

V = Total VOLUME to be infused in mL

T = Total TIME in minutes

C = Drop factor CALIBRATION (gtt/mL)

R = RATE of flow (gtt/min)

The short cut method to calculate IV flow rate is:

$$\frac{mL/h}{\text{Drop factor constant}} = \text{gtt/min}$$

Rules for IV Calculations—Infusion Time and Volume

To calculate IV infusion time:

$$\frac{\text{TOTAL volume}}{\text{mL/h}} = \text{TOTAL hours}$$

Use the flow rate formula to calculate time:

$$\frac{V}{T} \times C = R$$

"T" is the unknown.

To calculate IV volume:

$$\frac{V}{T} \times C = R$$

"V" is the unknown.

Rules for IV Calculations— Flow Rate, Safe Dosages, and IV PB

To calculate the flow rate (mL/h) for IV medications ordered in mg/min:

Step 1. Calculate dosage in (mL/min)

Step 2. Calculate the quantity to administer in mL/h

To check safe dosage of IV medications ordered in mL/h:

Step 1. Calculate mg/h

Step 2. Convert mg/h to mg/min

Follow these six steps to calculate the flow rate of an IV that includes IV PB. Calculate:

1. IV PB flow rate
2. Total IV PB time
3. Total IV PB volume
4. Total regular IV volume
5. Total regular IV time
6. Regular IV flow rate

Volume Control Set Review

■ Volume control sets have a drop factor of 60 gtt/mL.

■ The total volume of the medication, IV dilution fluid, and the IV flush fluid must be considered to calculate flow rates when using sets like Buretrol.

■ Use ratio-proportion to calculate flow rates for intermittent medications when a continuous IV rate in mL/h is prescribed.

Volume Control Set (Buretrol, Volutrol, or Soluset)

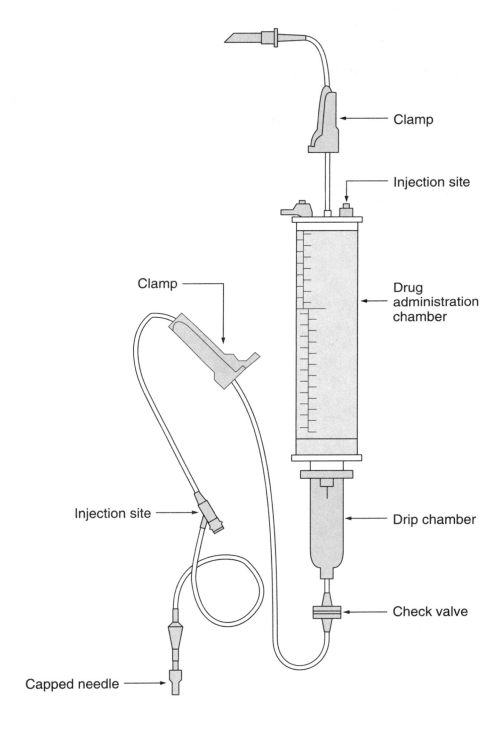

Clamp

Injection site

Clamp

Drug administration chamber

Injection site

Drip chamber

Check valve

Capped needle

Calculation of Daily Rate of Pediatric Maintenance IV Fluids

Use this formula to calculate the daily rate of pediatric maintenance IV fluids.

100 mL per kg per day for first 10 kg of body weight

50 mL per kg per day for next 10 kg of body weight

20 mL per kg per day for each kg of body weight above 20